Health Risks of Weight Loss

Frances M. Berg
Healthy Weight Journal

Published by *Healthy Weight Journal*
(formerly Obesity & Health),
Established in 1986
Healthy Living Institute
Editor: Frances M. Berg, M.S.
Associate Editor: Kendra Rosencrans, M.S.
Production Manager: Ronda Irwin.
Subscription rate: $59 per year (bimonthly)
Add $1 Canada; $9 other countries. U.S. funds only
Visa, MasterCard. Student and group rates available.
Healthy Weight Journal, Healthy Living Institute,
402 South 14th Street, Hettinger, ND, 58639
TE: 701-567-2646; FAX: 701-567-2602.

Contents

Contents

Introduction

The effects of the current obsession with dieting can be devestating. Pressures to be thin are more severe in the western world today than they have ever been in the past. These pressures – from television, Madison Avenue, magazines, Hollywood and the medical community – are so great that nearly half of American women and girls, and about one fourth of men, are actively trying to lose weight. These statistics include as many as 80 percent of girls as young as ten or 11 with disordered eating because of their fear of fat.

These facts prompt some disturbing questions.

Are these people – an estimated 60 to 80 million adults – improving their health by their weight loss efforts, or not? How safe are the methods they use? How does the drive to be thin and "always dieting" impact individuals of all sizes, their families and their communities?

Our obsession with weight and dieting is a national crisis not being adequately addressed by the health community. Significant rapid weight loss affects every part of the body, and can be fatal.

Since weight loss is a health-related endeavor, many might assume treatments are subject to clinical testing, accountability and regulation. Unfortunately, this is not the case. Even many medically supervised programs seem to proceed with the rationale that weight loss justifies any detrimental effects. High-risk patients are commonly subjected to high-risk treatments. Healthful solutions often do not get the attention or encouragement they deserve.

The powerful weight loss industry and its entrenchment with policy makers is undeniably partially responsible. Consumers spend $30 to $50 billion annually on weight loss services and products. This does not include smoking for weight control, which is a highly lucrative marketing area for the tobacco industry.

A dazzling array of weight loss methods is available – diet pills, surgery, exercise, starvation, purging, and a multitude of diets. They are heavily advertised, and promoted by friends, family and health professionals. Some interventions appear benign; others clearly entail risks much greater than the risks of overweight. Some are supervised by trained medical teams; others are self-administered by mere children.

Even repeated cycles of weight gain and loss, or simply weight loss itself in some degree, may be harmful. It is generally assumed that weight loss will improve the health of large people. But there is little research to support this.

Purpose of report

This report brings together the scientific evidence on the health risks of dieting and other weight loss interventions. It is intended to help both professionals and consumers cope in healthful ways with the complex dilemmas of weight. It is also intended to generate discussion which can lead to preventive action and a more comprehensive way of dealing with these issues.

The dangers of rapid, large weight loss must be recognized, short-term losses discouraged, and healthy weight guidelines encouraged. Consumers and professionals who understand the risks of succumbing to the latest fad diet or pill are better able to make sound decisions which promote good health.

Do diets work?

In the short term, weight loss treatment is often quite successful. In controlled settings, participants who remain in programs typically lose about 10 percent of their weight.

Traditionally, recommendations were for large people to lose weight until they reached "ideal weight." Maintenance was assumed. Few health professionals looked beyond those first few weeks of "success," and the patient was faulted for regain.

However, it has now become clear that lost weight is almost invariably regained. It is widely reported that 95 to 97 percent of weight loss efforts fail. There is little evidence in the scientific literature to refute this or to suggest any recent improvement. The involvement of vested interests in much of the research that is going on, without adequate controls, adds considerable confusion to study outcomes. Most treatment reports give only short-term results, which tend to show success, but may be quite irrelevant in the lifetime treatment of chronic diseases like diabetes.

Complex causes

The causes of obesity are not well understood.

The basic cause is believed to be an imbalance between calorie intake and energy expenditure. But food composition probably plays a role. High fat diets are linked to the development of obesity in laboratory animals even when calorie intake is the same.

The tendency to gain excessive weight varies from one person to another, even in the same family, and even when food intake, physical activity and lifestyle appear to be similar. It is possible that for some individuals, genetic factors may cause a greater amount of fat intake to be stored in the fat cells. These genetic factors may also protect stored fat, and work to restore fat after weight loss.

Research suggests that sedentary living and high-fat diets, and perhaps alcohol consumption, play important roles in the increasing prevalence of obesity throughout the world.

"In our society, there is a wide range of well-advertised and generally affordable foods, many of which are nutritionally unbalanced and highly caloric. This availability may encourage overeating. At the same time, our energy expenditure is diminished through sedentary lifestyles and the use of labor-saving devices at work and at home," explains the Task Force on the Treatment of Obesity, Health and Welfare Canada.

In the decades after the second world war, sedentary lifestyles became common at all age levels, and Americans began consuming a diet of about 42 percent fat and 25 percent sugar. Obesity rates rose accordingly, to 34 percent of U.S. adults.

Obesity increased even more rapidly for populations undergoing sudden culture change. This suggests the presence of a "thrifty gene" for people who formerly lived an extremely austere and active lifestyle.

Once considered a simple problem, easily solved, obesity is now recognized as a complex condition that resists intervention. Despite rapid advances, research in the field is quite recent. Disagreement and debate still prevail on nearly every key issue.

"Obesity continues to humble the scientific community by eluding effective understanding and intervention in many important respects," notes Shiriki Kumanyika, associate professor of nutrition epidemiology at Pennsylvania State University.

Considerable research suggests the body defends its normal weight through a highly regulated biological system. Fat cells both expand and multiply as more fat is gained. This effect and weight itself may be irreversible. The mechanisms which maintain and defend obesity probably include metabolism, hormones, fat cell storage, fat cell proliferation, appetite and satiety signals in the brain and digestive tract, and the rate of energy utilized in assimilating food and in physical activity. Psychological, social, economic and environmental factors may also be involved in the typical regain after weight loss.

Risks of weight

Statistics suggest apparent health risks associated with excess weight and fat distribution on the body.

Statistical risks and averages, however, apply to large groups and not necessarily to individuals. In a public health sense, the risks are critical because they affect large numbers of people. But the actual risks may in fact be small and likely to involve many complex factors. There is little reason to believe individuals cannot be healthy regardless of weight.

Overemphasizing obesity's health risks can increase stigma, worsen guilt and blame, increase social and medical pressures on persons of size, and increase employment and insurance difficulties.

Focusing on the risks also can increase fear of fat in the general population, exerting even more pressure on women, men and children to strive for excessive thinness. This in turn may promote eating disorders, dieting at ever younger ages, weight cycling, smoking for weight control, diet pill use and abuse, surgery, semi-starvation and nutritional deficiencies. This information can and is being abused and exploited to justify further discrimination and bigotry, and to sell harmful weight loss products and programs.

It is also important to realize that some negative health consequences attributed to obesity may in fact be the result of intense and repeated weight loss episodes. This possibility has not been widely recognized by the research community. Focusing on the risks of obesity without considering risks of intervention increases the likelihood of detrimental effects.

Looking ahead

The importance of these issues supports the urgency for weight to assume a high priority on the nation's health agenda. Viewing the "big picture," across the weight spectrum, reveals a complexity of problems.

This nation has not dealt well with weight issues in the past. Health policy has often been reactive to events in specific areas, rather than addressing real issues in a comprehensive way. Attempts to solve problems in one area have affected other areas adversely. The credo to "do no harm" is often abused in health care and in national policy.

Today educators and health care professionals are confronted with dilemmas like these:

- How can we prevent obesity, without increasing disordered eating, thinness obsession and size discrimination?
- How can we prevent eating disorders without increasing the prevalence of obesity?
- How can we help people manage their weight while honoring the credo to "do no harm"?
- How can we regulate and make accountable the large and diverse weight loss industry?

Many health professionals look for solutions to the development of safe and effective drugs, possibly 10 or 15 years away. While such drugs may be needed for some patients, there are ethical questions about how they will be used. Will they be used in longterm self-treatment by the general public? Will they be marketed to children?

Challenges

Challenges for the next decade are in these five areas:

- Attitude. Healthier attitudes will encompass an awareness and concern for the issues of weight, an acceptance of a wider range of shapes and sizes, and motivation to live healthy lifestyles.
- Lifestyle. Healthier lifestyles are a priority for people of all ages, stressing enjoyable activity, moderate lowfat eating, self-acceptance and positive relationships. Environmental changes are needed to encourage healthy lifestyles, rather than promoting obesity and eating disorders, as now.
- Health care. A fresh approach in health care is needed to enhance the health of large people instead of focusing on weight loss, which

has been unsuccessful. Regulation of the diet industry is needed to require accountability, and to insure that treatments are proven safe and effective before being marketed.

■ Prevention. Preventive efforts must have the three goals of improving lifestyles, decreasing dieting behavior and eating disorders, and preventing excess weight gain. They should be tested for safety and effectiveness, in the knowledge that the wrong kind of intervention can be worse than the problem.

■ Knowledge. Research needs span the health spectrum from genetic to biochemical, physiologic and neurophysiologic. We need to know more about the causes, treatment and prevention of obesity. Investigations focusing on both individuals and populations are needed, with particular emphasis on those most severely affected: minorities and women. Ethics in the treatment area, and better communication of research information to educators and health professionals are other critical areas. Consolidation of weight studies within one discipline would improve the possibility of dealing with issues in a comprehensive way.

Suggestions for today

Until more is known about safe and effective obesity treatment, appropriate advice for many larger persons may be to maintain a stable weight and avoid further weight gain.

The question of whether to treat or not to treat merits serious consideration. In Canada, where weight issues have received considerable national attention, health care workers are given a clear warning: If you cannot help, at least *do no harm.*

For persons with medical problems related to obesity, it appears that moderate, gradual weight loss may be beneficial if weight loss is maintained, and weight cycling avoided.

Whatever the decision, the focus must be improved health, not weight loss at any cost.

With this focus, weight goals may no longer be appropriate.

Instead, a conservative, moderate approach emphasizing permanent healthful lifestyle changes appears to be most beneficial. This may include increasing physical activity, decreasing fat consumption, increasing intake of fruits and vegetables, and decreasing or eliminating alcohol. Gradual and moderate changes which fit into one's current life situation are suggested. Extremes in exercise, eating patterns and food selection should be avoided.

Any weight lost this way, through habit change, is likely to be maintained. Whether weight is lost or not, the results are to be measured in terms of improved health and well-being.

- F. Berg

MISSION STATEMENT

As the leading journal in its field,
HEALTHY WEIGHT JOURNAL provides a critical link
between research and practical application.
Recognizing that weight is a complex condition of increasing
concern throughout the world, we are committed to
bringing together scientific information from many sources,
reporting controversial issues in a clear, objective manner,
and to the ongoing search for
truth and understanding.
Recognizing that weight is an easily exploitable
health and social concern, we are further
committed to exposing deception,
reshaping detrimental social attitudes, and
promoting good health at any size.
Our mission is to be a voice of integrity and insight in
a field that has been much abused and neglected.

PART I

RISKS
OF
WEIGHT
LOSS

1. General treatment risks

*"If you cannot help,
at least
do no harm."*
— Health and Welfare
Canada

Millions of Americans – children and adults, women and men – are trying to lose weight. Therefore, the consequences of dieting and weight loss have critical public health implications today.

Weight loss programs have never been more numerous – from medically monitored diets offered by clinics and hospitals to commercial diet centers to a host of other products and programs the dieter uses individually.

While there are responsible weight loss programs staffed by qualified professionals, many others represent what Rep. Ron Wyden, D-Ore., calls a "new mix of questionable products and untrained providers."

Obesity has health risks. But the quest for weight loss is also a risky venture, and those risks include injury and death from dieting, weight loss, and attempted weight loss.

Millions are dieting

Forty percent of women and 25 percent of men in the United States are trying to lose weight at any one time, according to a recent report by the Centers for Disease Control. Of these, 62 percent of women and 44 percent of men are not overweight according to their self-reported height and weight.[1]

Dieting among adolescents is even more prevalent. For some, dieting may almost be considered a way of life, says one researcher.

The CDC reports that 62 percent of girls and 28 percent of boys in grades 8 and 10 have been on a diet in the past year. Nearly 7 percent of adolescent girls are using diet pills. Among those who perceive them-

Figure 1

Dieting and purging
among high school students

	girls		boys	
Percent of total	White	Black	White	Black
Dieters	77%	61%	42%	41%
Liquid diet	14	24	6	9
Diet pills	23	16	6	0
Laxatives	7	18	5	2
Diuretics	5	11	1	2
Vomiting	16	3	7	0
Vomiting monthly or more often	8	1	-	-
Fasting monthly or more often	35	40	29	25

Dieting and inappropriate dieting behaviors are widely practiced by U.S. high school students. Total 1,269 students, Cleveland State University study.

HEALTHY WEIGHT JOURNAL(O&H)/CDC

selves as overweight, 23 percent vomit to reduce weight. Many potentially harmful dieting methods such as diet pills, laxatives, diuretics, vomiting and fasting *(Figure 1)*.

The CDC report warns that "harmful weight loss practices and negative attitudes about body size have been reported among girls as young as nine years of age."[2]

Dieting is closely linked to disordered eating behaviors. Some investigators consider dieting to be a necessary factor in the development of eating disorders.

An estimated 10 percent of U.S. high school and college students have eating disorders, 90 to 95 percent of them female. By some estimates .2 to 1 percent have anorexia nervosa and 1 to 3 percent bulimia nervosa, both potentially fatal.

Weight is a major issue for young athletes in sports such as wrestling and gymnastics. Many high school wrestlers use extreme fluid and food deprivation in their efforts to "make weight" for a match. Concerns have been raised about their dehydration, possible delayed growth and development during a period of active growth, initiation of eating disorders, and short term effects including weakness, cold intolerance and lack of concentration.[3]

"A new mix of questionable products, untrained providers and deceptive advertising is exposing our citizens to unexpected health risks."
— Rep. Ron Wyden

Treatment methods

Weight loss interventions include a confusing array of treatment programs and products, such as:

- Surgery: gastric bypass, vertical banded gastroplasty, other types, numerous versions
- Liposuction, tummy tuck
- Jaw wiring, gastric balloon
- Very low calorie diet, fasting
- Low and moderately low calorie diet
- Behavior modification
- Drugs and diet pills which are claimed to speed metabolism, suppress appetite and/or block digestion
- Laxatives and diuretics
- Smoking
- Meal supplements
- Weight loss centers providing diet and various combinations of exercise, supplements, products
- Hypnotism
- Body wraps
- Spot reducers, creams and lotions
- Herbal treatments
- Acupuncture
- Passive exercise machines, electrical stimulators
- Exercise and exercise equipment

Many of these are considered radical and potentially dangerous

methods that require careful medical monitoring – which often is not provided. Responsible programs operate alongside fraudulent ones. Too many exaggerate their safety and success claims.

Diets and diet products frequently are self-administered by the consumer, who may be age 9 or younger, according to a recent study.

Information about the safety and effectiveness of diet products and programs is unavailable, said Wyden, who chaired the congressional subcommittee that investigated the weight loss industry in 1990.[4] Statistics on dropout rates, how much patients typically lose during treatment, how many gain back the weight and how soon, and short- and long-term adverse health effects are also unavailable, he said. "It is unconscionable that so many questions remain unanswered."

Wyden said 65 million Americans are affected by being overweight or thinking they're overweight, and most are willing to try anything to lose weight.

C. Wayne Callaway, an associate clinical professor of medicine at George Washington University, testified at the hearings as a physician and on behalf of the American Board of Nutrition.[5]

Nearly a century of scientific information exists that explains the changes which occur in response to low calorie and very low calorie diets, Callaway said.

"With rare exceptions, none of the popular commercially available programs for treating obesity is based on current scientific knowledge." If they were, they could no longer promise rapid weight loss, he said.

Callaway said the lack of properly trained professionals in the weight loss industry is a concern. "Supervision of such programs varies from none, to instantly created 'certified counselors,' to physicians with little or no training in this area, to a few physicians and registered dietitians and behavioral psychologists who truly have the required expertise."

High-risk programs

The Canadian Task Force on the Treatment of Obesity gives the following warning about three types of programs:[6]

■ **Nutritionally deficient programs.** It must be assumed that diets of less than 1,200 calories per day based on regular foods will not provide sufficient vitamins, minerals and nutrients to meet an individual's requirements. Nonetheless, these diets are being used in some treatment programs, without the necessary supervision of physicians and dietitians.

■ **Diets less than 900 calories.** Very low calorie diets should be provided only under medical supervision by a doctor specially trained to treat obesity, working with an interdisciplinary team of health professionals. This may not always be the case at present.

■ **Medications.** Both oral and injected medications, which are ineffective – and for some persons potentially harmful – are being used in some weight-reduction programs. Neither human chorionic gonadotrophin nor vitamin injections, per se, are effective in inducing weight loss, and unless administered to treat some known deficiency, their use touches on possible malpractice.

Dexfenfluramine use risks brain damage

A diet drug under consideration by the Food and Drug Administration could put patients at risk for brain damage, says a Johns Hopkins University researcher. At the center of the controversy is the drug dexfenfluramine, widely used in Europe.

Neurologist George Ricaurte exposed monkeys to the drug and reported finding evidence of damage in brain cells whose function it is to process serotonin, a brain chemical that helps regulate mood, sleep, aggression, appetite and impulse control. He said the damage is demonstrated by showing the level of serotonin is reduced in one part of the serotonin neuron.

Under FDA review are 18 dexfenfluramine studies involving more than 4,000 patients. Approval is requested by Interneuron Pharmaceuticals of Lexington, MA. *(AP 1994)*[81]

Big business

Obesity intervention is a health-related procedure.

But it is also big business. Numerous charges have been leveled recently – through Congressional hearings, the New York City Consumer Affairs Office, federal and state regulatory agencies, Health and Welfare Canada, and independent consumer groups – that business frequently gets in the way of health and safety.

Americans spent $30.2 billion dollars on weight loss in 1990, according to Marketdata, a Valley Stream, N.Y., marketing analysis firm.[7] This is in addition to the estimated $5 to $6 billion spent on fraudulent weight loss products, and an unknown amount spent on surgery.

The U.S. Center for Health Statistics estimated spending at $30 to $50 billion in 1994.

These estimates don't include the billions spent on the tobacco industry, which is closely involved in weight issues, or mainline cosmetic firms which have recently moved into questionable areas such as marketing treatments for "cellulite."

These powerful industries have a vested interest in keeping public attention focused on the very thin cultural ideal, an obsession with weight, and the health risks of obesity.

Their activities are highly visible through advertising, programming and editorial decisions. They are also intimately involved in funding research at prestigious institutions, and are involved in presentations at conferences and reports published in the scientific literature.

The weight loss industry has been assumed to be harmless.

But three congressional hearings held in 1990 by the U.S. House Subcommittee on Regulation, Business Opportunities and Energy showed that it is not. Testimony before the subcommittee described the severe injuries and tragedies caused by diet programs.

Questioning assumptions

The hearings exposed, for the first time, what was going on in the diet industry, and raised questions about whether consumers were being treated fairly. Chaired by Wyden, the hearings revealed widespread abuse in the weight loss industry. The findings forced reluctant regulatory agencies, such as the Food and Drug Administration and the Federal Trade Commission, to take action against fraud and false advertising in the weight loss industry.[8]

The hearings were followed by a major National Institutes of Health Technology Assessment Conference in 1992 on evaluating Methods for Voluntary Weight Loss and Control. After two days of testimony, the conference panel issued a statement reporting that:

- Weight loss strategies have caused harm.
- Most often weight lost is regained.
- Dropout rates are high.
- Repeated lose and gain cycles may have adverse effects.
- Trying to achieve body weights and shapes presented in the media is not an appropriate goal for most people.
- Unrealistically thin ideals are a problem.
- Many Americans who are not overweight are trying to lose weight and this may have significant physical and psychological health consequences.

Americans spend $30 to $50 billion dollars on weight loss – not including surgery, an estimated $5 to $6 billion for fraudulent products, or cigarettes.

● Most major studies suggest that increased mortality is associated with weight loss.

This was a landmark statement in the obesity field. For the first time leaders in the health community showed a readiness to question long-held assumptions about weight loss.

Adverse effects

Until very recently it was assumed that weight loss by any means is beneficial for overweight individuals. Radical methods were prescribed with the rationale that weight loss justifies nearly any detrimental effects, particularly since many very large persons have health risks.

It was further assumed that everyone can succeed in weight loss and that most commercial programs are safe and effective.

These assumptions are by no means valid today.

The Michigan Health Council Task Force to Establish Weight Loss Guidelines cites these potentially negative effects of weight loss:[9]

■ Health complications from the weight-loss process, such as cardiac arrhythmias, hypokalemia, hyperuricemia, gallbadder damage and death.

■ Psychological damage, such as depression and diminishment of self-esteem from repeated "failure" at weight loss.

■ Initiation of binge eating and eating disorders following semi-starvation regimens.

■ Long-term complications and indirect ill effects.

■ Damage from weight-cycling, repeated weight loss and regain.

Janet Polivy, PhD, a professor of psychology and psychiatry at the University of Toronto, who has researched dieting and its effects for over 16 years, documents the following health complications directly attributed to weight loss:[10]

● gallstones

● cardiac disorders

● fainting, weakness and fatigue

● both slowed and increased heart rate

● elevated cholesterol

● anemia

● gouty arthritis

● edema

● headache

● nausea

● hair loss and thinning hair

● hypotension

● diarrhea, constipation

● aching muscles

● abdominal pain

● elevated uric acid levels

● cold intolerance

● loss of lean tissue

"After seven weeks on a 1,000-calorie diet, Mike had a full cardiac arrest, went into a six-day coma . . . and will never work independently again."

- changes in liver function
- dry skin
- muscle cramps
- amenorrhea and decreased libido
- refeeding complications from fasting diets such as edema, potassium deficiencies, biliary tract disorders, pancreatic complications
- death

The classic starvation study, conducted at the University of Minnesota in 1944-1945, documents these and other changes that take place under conditions of semi-starvation.[11] Many of the physical and emotional changes observed for the 32 volunteers in the wartime study are experienced today by individuals on restrictive diets. The study is published in *The Biology of Human Starvation,* by Ancel Keys.

Even exercising can be harmful, the Michigan Task Force warned, particularly for overweight persons not accustomed to being active. For some people physical exertion can entail health risks; for others it can be dangerous under certain conditions. Clients should be screened for conditions which could make exercise hazardous and, if at risk, monitored for abnormal responses during exercise.[12]

Radical methods are prescribed with the rationale that weight loss justifies nearly any detrimental effects.

Consumer incidents

At the 1990 congressional hearings, three individuals testified as victims or on behalf of victims of the weight loss industry who had developed severe medical complications related to the program they had followed.

One woman, who remained unidentified, told about her husband, Mike, who before going on Nutri/System, was a successful college professor with a doctorate in engineering. In 1985, after seven weeks on a 1,000-calorie diet prescribed by the program, Mike had a full cardiac arrest and went into a six-day coma. His heart had weakened as the result of a potassium and protein deficiency which his doctor believed were related to his diet, she reported. Mike's doctor indicated his potassium shortage likely caused his heart's electrical impulse to falter, and his weakened heart muscle couldn't resume beating, she said.

A week prior to the cardiac arrest, Mike had complained of feeling light-headed after exercising and had passed out for a few moments. When he discussed the incident with the nurse at the weight loss center, she told him to eat more fruit.

Doctors later discovered signs of heart disease. "Our cardiac physician suggested that if Mike had been properly evaluated by a physician he most likely would not have been recommended for a non-medically supervised diet," the woman said.

Unfortunately, he never fully recovered. "Mike will never work independently again and his daily activities must be planned and supervised," she said. "He has no technical knowledge. He cannot initiate intellectual conversation. He's often confused and forgets current information. I have become his caretaker and protector."

Sherri Steinberg of Coral Springs, Fla., also testified to problems with a commercial diet program. One night about two months into the

"The lights went out in our lives on July 12, 1989, when our beautiful, fun-loving, and soon-to-be-married daughter, Noelle (died) of cardiac arrest."

diet and after losing 28 pounds, Steinberg suddenly "doubled over in excruciating pain" and was rushed to the emergency room. Her gallbladder was removed a few days later.

"I've still never fully recovered," Steinberg said. "The (counselors) never told me any of this could happen."

Children rarely develop gallstones, but a 13-year-old girl also had to have her gallbladder removed after losing weight through a diet prescribed by the Doctor's Quick Weight Loss Center. Her mother, Loretta Pameijer, testified that her daughter was given a cursory physical plus a test for food allergies before beginning the program. Then she was given a food chart that supposedly reflected the allergy test results and listed foods the girl could and couldn't eat.

Although her daughter followed the diet faithfully, there were times when she would stop losing weight, Pameijer said. "The counselors would put her on a 'parsley break.' It had almost nothing in it but meat and a half a cup of parsley a day."

The girl's physician said she had "the worst gallbladder attack" he had ever seen in anyone so young.

"We're angry because it never occurred to us to be suspicious of a doctor's clinic," Pameijer said.

A bereaved father testified at the hearings, protesting the easy availability of diet pills at groceries, discount outlets and corner drug stores. "The lights went out in our lives on July 12, 1989, when our beautiful, fun-loving, and soon-to-be-married daughter, Noelle (died) of cardiac arrest. These stores have no more business selling these drugs to children than they do liquor to a minor."

He read from a friend's letter: "Noelle told me while we were in college together in 1988 that her use of diet pills had accelerated to as many as 8 to 10 boxes a week. She complained of poor concentration and admitted to feeling nervous and irritable. She said she could not afford diet pills, but confessed to stealing Dexatrim and Acutrim on occasion, and borrowed money when possible to support her abuse. I believe the availability and easy access to diet pills, laxatives and diuretics was a major contributing factor to her eating disorder which led to her tragic death."

Another young woman testified, "My eating disorder stole my teen years . . . It ripped apart my life. I took whole boxes of diet pills at a time. I would get weak, dizzy, nauseous and I even passed out. I knew something was wrong, but in spite of everything, I continued to take pills and lose weight. I hope Congress will act soon to help get diet pills off the shelves."

The New York investigation also turned up numerous cases of injury. One 39-year-old Brooklyn woman lost her gallbladder after six months on a Nutri/System program. She said she didn't know she was endangering her health when she signed up to lose 69 pounds, but after subsisting for three months solely on the pre-packaged food, she began to feel ill and complained of stomach and upper chest pains to her counselors. "They said don't worry about it," she recalled. "They walked around in white lab coats, but they never had real doctors there."

Unfortunately, this was not an isolated case, said the investigators, but one of 30 New York diet victims suing the company. In one of the cases, a 15-year-old Long Island girl had her gallbladder removed after a six-month rapid weight loss of 72 pounds.

Callaway says the company claim that obesity – not dieting – is the major cause of gallbladder disease comes "more than a decade after the association between dieting and gallstones was first recognized. And it comes nearly a year after a study in the *Archives of Internal Medicine*, showed that in eight weeks of dieting on a 500 calorie diet, 25 percent of dieters developed gallstones. In contrast, equally overweight individuals who did not diet showed no development of gallstones during that brief eight week interval."

Fast weight loss promotes gallstones

Gallstones form up to 15 to 25 times faster for persons on very low calorie diets over the general obese population, according to University of Alabama nutrition researchers. They find new stones form in 10 to 26 percent of persons on VLCDs and may occur within four weeks. Their report says the stones produce symptoms in about one-third of the subjects, and about half of these undergo surgery. They warn that this may have great impact on public health and demands on health care facilities.

The three factors they suggest as being involved in increased gallstone risk are: calorie level, rate of weight loss, and duration of treatment. Very low calorie levels and rapid weight loss are associated with increased risk, and longer periods of rapid weight loss with more risk than shorter periods.

Obesity itself is associated with increased bile stasis and cholesterol saturation, and an increased risk of gallstones, say the Alabama researchers. Weight loss can improve this by normalizing bile composition. However, they warn that the process of weight loss needs more study.

The Alabama researchers ask, what is a medically safe rate of weight loss to avoid gallstone formation?

From a literature review, they advise that weight loss should not exceed an average of 3.3 pounds (1.5 kg) per week. At higher rates, gallstone formation rises to 1.6 to 3.2 percent of subjects per week. At lower weight loss levels the risk is 0 to 0.5 percent of subjects per week.

Gallstone formation apparently is not affected by the diet's fat content. Rather, in their studies, it was linked to the rate of weight loss or degree of calorie restriction.

Since the effects of gradual weight loss on gallstone formation are unknown, the researchers urge this be investigated in the interests of safety of weight reduction programs. They also suggest further studies on the effect of the weight loss process on fat content, refeeding effects, and the mechanisms underlying the etiology of cholelithiasis.[13]

Gallstones cost $5 billion

Gallstones are the most common and the most costly digestive disease with an estimated annual cost of more than $5 billion. They are more prevalent in women who have had multiple pregnancies, are obese, or who have experienced rapid weight loss, as well as among older patients and certain ethnic groups, says the consensus statement of the National Institutes of Health published after the September 1992 Conference on Gallstones and Laparoscopic Cholecystectomy.

The conference found that more than 20 million Americans have gallstones. In the past two years the new laparoscopic cholecystectomy procedure has shortened what was a five-day hospital stay, along with

"We don't know how many are dying."
– Janet Polivy

In eight weeks of dieting on a 500 calorie diet, 25 percent of dieters, developed gallstones.

decreasing costs, pain and scarring.[14]

Dieting deaths

Health risks associated with low calorie diets have been the subject of debate since the 1970s, when the documented deaths of 58 persons on liquid protein diets, and six deaths in the early 1980s from the Cambridge diet caused a diet scandal.[15]

Medical experts agree that current formula diets are better than the old formulas, says the New York report. But "what the diet companies themselves do know is that health complications if not fatalities are possible with their diets. It is impossible to know if sudden deaths are still occurring since there is currently no mechanism for tracking diet-related deaths."

"We don't know how many are dying," warns Polivy.

During weight loss, the body uses its own fat reserves, the report explains, but if weight loss is too rapid, the body will also draw from lean mass. When this happens, muscle and organ tissue are gradually lost, damage that can affect the heart.

The British COMA report warns that rapid weight loss of up to 2 kg per week can only be achieved at the expense of non-fat tissues. The more rapid the rate of weight loss, the greater the proportion of lean tissue loss, which is generally considered to be undesirable. Loss of lean tissue can disturb cardiac function and damage other organs, according to obesity specialists.[16]

A recent report in the *Journal of the American Medical Association* by a group of physicians long experienced in prescribing VLCDs[17] warned of the diet's hazards. Specifically, they warned of use by untrained physicians and medically unsupervised use.

The Michigan Task Force lists sudden and potentially fatal cardiac arrhythmias (prolonged QT interval, ventricular fibrillation, multifocal premature ventricular contractions, and atrial fibrillation) as risks of diets with less than 800 calories. Other potential side effects of very low calorie diets are listed in the Michigan Task Force guidelines, *Toward Safe Weight Loss.*[18] The report recommends VLCDs be used only in a strictly supervised hospital setting and only when the consequences of obesity are a greater life threat than the risks of the diet.

Such diets are commonly prescribed for both high-risk and low-risk patients and often last 12 to 16 weeks or more. A very low calorie diet should not last more than four weeks, according to the British COMA recommendations.

Curiously, one of the medical criteria for rapid weight loss programs is that only heavier patients should be accepted (130 percent or more of desirable weight) – those who may be at highest risk. One explanation is that lower weight people may lose too much lean mass. But this does not explain why high-risk persons should be treated with high-risk, rapid weight loss programs.

Nancy Wellman, PhD, President of the American Dietetic Association, warns that, "the most significant drawback to these diets is the potential for life-threatening side effects . . . The loss of body protein – and here we are talking about muscle tissue – may affect cardiac function and could be related to heart failure."

United Weight Control Corp., a medically supervised fasting program investigated by the New York Consumer Affairs Office, acknowl-

The Michigan Task Force lists sudden and potentially fatal cardiac arrhythmias as risks of diets with less than 800 calories.

edges the risk of sudden death in the "tiny type" of an informed consent contract that dieters are required to sign when they begin the program. It reads:

"Some reports have suggested a relationship between programmed diets and sudden death, probably due to irregularities of the heart. I understand that participation in this weight reduction program may entail a minute risk of fatal heart irregularities."

At the 1990 congressional hearing, Callaway from George Washington University testified that sudden deaths are still occuring from current liquid formula diets. "The fact that we have not heard about them until recently reflects our lack of any type of tracking mechanism. We have no way of knowing how common these occurances are.

"When the victim or her survivors have raised legal issues, the cases have generally been settled out of court and the documents sealed. There is no registry for providing data on a national scale and, as you can well appreciate, the companies themselves do not volunteer such information to outside researchers. It is only when media attention is brought to bear on this problem, as occurred with the extremely high frequence of gallstones in people on low calorie diets, that victims recognize that they are not simply isolated cases," he said.

VLCDs are associated with 59 sudden deaths per 100,000, according to Lars Sjostrom, University of Goteborg, in Goteborg, Sweden.[19]

Sjostrom says the relationship between sudden death, body weight and obesity intervention is complex.

He cites a study by E. Drenick and J. Fisler in which sudden death (cardiac arrest unexplained by autopsy) has a frequency of 1.6 per 100,000 women annually in the general population.[20] But in 60 cases of sudden deaths among 50,314 morbidly obese surgery patients followed by 144 obesity surgeons for an average 22 months, the estimated annual mortality in sudden death was 65 per 100,000, 40 times higher than expected. The relation to rapid weight loss is not clear because eight of the patients in the surgical material died while waiting for surgery, says Sjostrom.

The figure is close to the annual rate of 59 sudden deaths per 100,000 patients on liquid formula diets, he points out.

He expresses hope that the Swedish Obese Subjects study (SOS), a controlled, long-term study of 7,000 to 10,000 obese persons throughout Sweden investigating the effects of treating obesity, will provide some answers on the risk reversibility in postobese subjects.[21]

Sjostrom reports that a Finnish study found no relationship between sudden death and weight for 3,589 men age 40 to 59 at entry, followed for 11 years. The Framingham study found a positive relationship between sudden death and weight for men without prior coronary heart disease, but the opposite for men with the disease, and no relationship for women.

It is ironic that most deaths are blamed on the victims' overweight, rather than the true culprit – radical attempts to lose weight, says Polivy, the University of Toronto professor of psychology and psychiatry.

Canada set new guidelines for health professionals in the wake of publicity surrounding the death of a woman in the lobby of a Toronto building that housed the diet center she attended.

Health and Welfare Canada warns that agressive treatment for weight loss can result in life-threatening complications. "Policy makers must be absolutely sure that strategies will improve individual well-

"Victims recognize they are not simply isolated cases – only when media attention is brought to bear on this problem."

Gastric reduction surgery
for severe obesity
is associated with a
1 percent death rate.
— *AMA DATTA panel*

being."[12] The guidelines warn professionals that their cardinal principle in weight strategy must be: "If you cannot help, at least do no harm."

The inquest into the Toronto woman's death determined that it was her dieting on a 900-calorie regimen, along with diuretics and diet pills prescribed by her medical doctor, that caused her death by heart attack.

Dieting deaths are not recorded in U.S. mortality statistics, according to the Centers for Disease Control in Atlanta. Reporting is not required and there is no surveillance of dieting programs. Most deaths associated with dieting appear to be listed as cardiac arrest.

Even if it were mandated by law, establishing a registry for recording deaths related to dieting would be difficult says F. Xavier Pi-Sunyer, of the Obesity Research Center in New York.

Such deaths are "very difficult to pin down, unless the family does something, and then it may be settled out of court."

When there is a death of someone on a very low calorie diet, he says, neither the physician nor the hospital want it publicized. They have a stake in wanting adverse effects to appear as natural causes. Many of these are high-risk patients, and it can be suggested the patient would have had a heart attack whether on the diet or not.

Among chronic cases of anorexia nervosa, one study found 7 percent of patients, mostly young women, had died within 10 years. Another found a death rate of 20 percent in 30 years. It is estimated that about 1 percent of American high school and college girls have anorexia nervosa.[22]

The death rate from gastric bypass surgery and vertical-banded gastroplasty, the two most common stomach reduction surgeries for severe obesity, was estimated at 1 percent in 1989 by the American Medical Association Diagnostic and Therapeutic Assessment panel (DATTA) which studied their safety and effectiveness. Surgery specialists suggest that the rate is lower than average at major institutions doing large numbers of gastric surgeries, and higher for smaller hospitals and surgical practices.[23]

Sudden death syndrome continues to chill treatment centers

Even though dieting deaths have been kept quiet since the rash of deaths in the 1970s, they are still occurring, warn researchers at the National Institutes of Health Obesity Research Center at St. Luke's-Roosevelt Hospital in New York.

"Sudden deaths during dieting continue," report Steven Heymsfield and Dympna Gallagher. "Over the past decade our group has reviewed the records of a number of unpublished litigation cases that fit the classical pattern of dietary-associated prolonged QTc interval and sudden death."[24]

They caution that vigorous weight loss should no longer be advocated for high-risk patients, due to evidence it may be associated both with sudden death and increased mortality.

Women appear more predisposed to the sudden death syndrome than men, they report, although statistics are unknown.

The researchers say the highest risk for sudden death syndrome is:
● during weight loss with total
   fasting

- during very low calorie diets
- following obesity surgery

Death may occur during rapid or prolonged weight loss, or in some cases during refeeding. Sudden death or syncope may follow what appears to be relatively minor stressful situations.

Typically the patient was in reasonably good health before treatment.

Two heart abnormalities usually identified when an electrocardiogram is available are: a reduction in the QRS complex amplitude, and QT interval prolongation after correction for heart rate. Autopsy shows a decreased heart size relative to pre-treatment body weight. Coronary arteries are patent and no abnormalities are present in valves or related structures.

Causes of death unknown

Sudden death syndrome remains unexplained, but Gallagher and Heymsfield suggest these theories:
- nutritionally inadequate diets
- depletion of myocardial proteins
- excessive B-adrenergic sensitivity of the myocardium
- electrolyte abnormalities
- ingestion of prescription medications that increase the risk of arrhythmia
- the presence of inherited defects that predispose to arrhythmias

Janis Fisler, PhD, Division of Cardiology, UCLA, Los Angeles, has investigated sudden death in starvation, very-low-calorie dieting and gastric surgery for the past decade and reports that heart irregularities, nutrition deficiencies and stress may be involved in the inconsistencies found in the syndrome.[25]

The heart is usually small and atrophic in children or adults who die of protein-calorie malnutrition or anorexia, even though it may actually be a larger portion of body weight in the starved than in control subjects, says Fisler. She cites a study that showed a 21 percent decline in heart weight for obese men who lost 27 percent of body weight after gastric surgery.

Left ventricular dysfunction is present to some extent in weight-reduced subjects, she reports. Low voltage, QTc prolongation and bradycardia are consistent findings in adult starvation. Another therapeutic starvation study of 13 subjects showed low voltage by week 7, prolongation of QT corrected for heart rate by week 8, eventual abnormality in seven subjects (Pringle). One patient in the weight loss program had two cardiac arrests.

Fisler says the five to seven week trials cited to prove safety may be too short to show adverse effects. Significant voltage change or QTc prolongation may not develop until after seven to eight weeks of caloric restriction.

Deficiencies on starvation or semistarvation diets may include lack of high-quality protein, electrolytes, or minerals such as potassium, magnesium and copper, she says.

Stress also may be a factor. Sudden death is preceded by acute psychological disturbances in 20 to 40 percent of cases, she explains. Syncope after stress and sudden death are known hazards in the presence of QT interval prolongation. The long QT syndrome, a consistent finding in sudden death during starvation or semistarvation diets, and ventricular arrhythmias can occur with strong psychological stress such as strong emotions or loud noise.

Anxiety, rapid weight loss, shifts in fluid or electrolyte homeostasis, surgical trauma and physical exertion, for example, may cause stress and, secondarily, autonomic imbalance. A subset of patients with QT interval prolongation would then be prone to unpredictable acute arrhythmias. Fisler says the clustering of deaths in the immediate pre-and postoperative period in her study with Drenick suggests that stress evoked autonomic imbalance leading to these deaths.[26]

Nutrition, stress may trigger syndrome

Fisler proposes the following explanation for the sudden cardiac deaths which are occurring due to severe caloric restriction:

"Obesity leads to myocardial hypertrophy and ECG abnormalities, including a prolonged QTc interval. Rapid and/or major weight loss damages the heart by decreasing myocardial fiber size. Lack of protein, electrolytes, and micronutrients may contribute to the myofibrillar damage. As a result of this damage, electrical instability occurs because of regional inhomogeneities in conduction or generation of abnormal impulses. Transient extra cardiac stimuli, including stress, alter sympathetic nervous system activity, and catecholamines, acting upon the electrically unstable heart, may precipitate fatal arrhythmias.

"This hypothesis implies that no single nutritional deficiency needs to be invoked as the cause of the arrhythmias and may explain the inconsistent findings in the cases of sudden death reported."

Earlier, at the end of the 1992 conference on Methods for Voluntary Weight Loss and Control, NIH issued a warning: "For most weight loss methods, there are few scientific studies evaluating their effectiveness and safety . . . The lack of data is especially disconcerting in view of the large number of Americans trying to lose weight . . . Commercial weight loss programs should routinely compile data on participant characteristics, attrition rates, degree and duration of weight loss, and adverse effects for all participants."

Gallagher and Heymsfield say the risk of sudden death syndrome is probably not high, or the resultant publicity would likely have uncovered an "epidemic" of cases during the peak of very-low-calorie dieting in the late 1980s.

However, researchers agree there is almost no information available on the sudden death syndrome and the statistics surrounding it. Most patients appear unaware of their risks for sudden death syndrome in restrictive dieting. Unless there are lawsuits that establish a public record (usually settled quietly out of court), and diligent investigative work, mortality statistics will continue to be obscured.

Heymsfield says he would like to see all deaths during very low calorie diets be designated as reportable deaths to the Centers of Disease Control.

Most patients appear unaware of their risks for sudden death syndrome in restrictive dieting.

2. Starvation and fad diets

Starvation and semi-starvation diets carry health risks, even when medically monitored. The risks escalate when individuals engage in their own fasting, fad diets and liquid diets without medical supervision.

Yet, despite the high risk of these diets, they have often been prescribed for high-risk patients. The rationale has been that patients with risk factors for chronic disease need to lose weight rapidly to reduce these risk factors, no matter what the cost may be to their health.

Often that cost has been too high.

Very low calorie diets

The modern very low calorie diet, or VLCD, usually consists of a liquid formula of 800 calories or less per day, sometimes as low as 300 calories. Examples are Optifast, Medifast and New Directions.

The modern VLCD formula is a high quality, animal-based protein, with little or no carbohydrate or fat. A second, less-used form uses solid animal foods – meat, poultry and fish. Also made of high quality protein, with little carbohydrate or fat, this version has been called the "protein-sparing-fast," because of an unsubstantiated theory by its promoters that it spares muscle tissue while reducing fat.

In Britain, the 1987 COMA Report of the United Kingdom Department of Health recommended that the VLCD be limited to no longer than four weeks because of its high risk. This report said the diet should provide at least 400 calories per day, and that losses of more than 1 to 2.2 pounds per week may be undesirable because of the increased loss of lean muscle tissue.

There are no such standards in the United States. VLCDs are commonly prescribed for 12 to 16 weeks and sometimes much longer. Weight losses can be enormous. One man in Oregon lost over 300 pounds in just over a year (25 pounds a month), dropping from 506 pounds to less than 205. A 500-pound woman in Cape Town lost 288 pounds in 18 months.[1] However, most loses range from 40 to 80 pounds.

The modern VLCD is an outgrowth of the zero calorie diet of the 1950s, the Metrecal craze of the early 1960s and the liquid protein diets of the 1970s and early 1980s.

Deaths associated with VLCDs have been reported for more than 25 years. Fifty-eight people died from liquid protein diets in the 1970s, and six deaths were documented in the early 1980s from the Cambridge liquid diet. The Food and Drug Administration reported 17 deaths occurred after two to six months on a liquid protein diet containing collagen, a low-quality protein.[2]

VLCDs produce rapid and significant results, but experts agree that long term results are poor. Most patients quickly regain their lost weight.

Michigan: toward safe weight loss

Risks of VLCDs may vary with the individual and the diet composition. The Michigan Health Council warns of the following potential risks:

■ **Cardiac arrhythmias:** Prolonged QT interval, ventricular fibrillation,

Deaths associated with very low calorie diets have been reported for more than 25 years.

VLCD destroys self-initiative

Enthusiasm for the very low calorie diet (VLCD) rests largely on the belief that VLCD will produce rapid weight loss. Of course, this is so (when) there are substantial losses of body water, but weight loss of this sort is not sustained, nor would it be desirable if it were.

It has been argued that the initial rapid weight loss on VLCD motivates patients to keep to the diet, which they would not have done with conventional diets. I know of no evidence to support this, and our experience is that compliance is similar in outpatients on either VLCD or conventional diets.

The "benefit" is slightly more rapid loss of the first 20 kg, but the penalties in my view, outweigh this.

The commercial basis for these diets makes it necessary to undermine the faith of obese patients in conventional diets. This attitude is reinforced, for commercial reasons, by counsellors. The patient is trained to become dependent on the physician, rather than learning independence, which is necessary for long-term weight maintenance.

VLCD is not needed by the severely obese patient (because everyone would lose weight on a conventional diet), and still less by the mildly obese patient, but it is needed by diet manufacturers and physicians associated with commercial weight loss organizations.

The cost in time and money of the diet, the clinic attendances and the laboratory tests is far greater with VLCD.

The net effect is that obese people are put to additional expense to buy a product that they do not need, and their confidence in their ability to control their own diet is unnecessarily destroyed.[s1]

– John Garrow, MD, Medical College of St. Bartholomew's Hospital, London.

multifocal premature ventricular contractions, and atrial fibrillation have all been observed. Arrhythmias can occur suddenly, without warning, and are potentially fatal.

■ **Inability to maintain long-term weight loss:** Rapid and/or repeated weight loss may slow basal metabolic rate, reducing calories needed. Lost weight may be regained quickly, and be more difficult to lose again in the future. Depression and diminished self-esteem are likely sequelae to weight regain.

■ **Initiation of binge eating:** The event initiating the development of anorexia and bulimia is almost invariably severe calorie restriction.

■ **Emotional changes:** VLCDs have been associated with emotional withdrawal, depression, anxiety and irritability.

■ **Loss of body protein:** Muscle and organ tissue is gradually lost with extreme caloric deprivation.

■ **Dehydration:** VLCDs, particularly if low in carbohydrate, can induce excessive diuresis, leading to decreased blood volume, which can lead to postural hypotension. Dehydration is potentially fatal.

■ **Ketosis:** VLCDs, particularly if low in carbohydrate, can cause ketosis. Ketosis is widely believed to cause euphoria and decreased appetite, although not all researchers agree. Ketosis can interfere with concentration and cause strong, unpleasant breath and body odor. In extreme cases may lower blood pH, which can be fatal. Ketosis is hazardous for pregnant women and insulin-dependent diabetics. Can be avoided if carbohydrate and calorie levels are high enough.

■ **Hypoglycemia:** VLCDs can result in excessively low levels of glucose in the blood, which may cause headaches, fatigue, inability to concentrate, sleepiness and cardiac arrhythmias.

■ **Hypokalemia:** VLCDs can result in excessively low levels of potassium in the blood, which may lead to cardiac arrhythmias.

■ **Hyperuricemia:** Excess uric acid levels have been caused by VLCDs. Gouty arthritis or uric acid kidney stones may be caused or exacerbated.

■ **Fibrosis of vital organs:** An abnormal increase in fibrous connective tissue in the organs may occur with repeated attempts at weight loss using starvation methods.

■ **Hair loss:** Hair loss is a well-documented side effect of VLCDs; usually temporary.

■ **Anemia:** VLCDs have been associated with anemia, characterized by fatigue, lassitude, weakness, pallor, reduced resistance to infection, lowered exercise tolerance and decreased attention span.

■ **Re-feeding edema:** With very low carbohydrate diets, large amounts of water may be retained when carbohydrates are consumed in a re-feeding process.

■ **Other documented side effects:** Included in other side effects are constipation or diarrhea, headaches, nausea, dry skin, gallstones, muscle cramps, bad breath, fatigue, cold intolerance, menstrual irregularities, and transient skin rash.

The Michigan Health Council Task Force developed the warnings at the height of VLCD popularity in 1989 in response to health concerns about the "potentially-dangerous practices in the weight loss industry."[3] The state had earlier documented seven deaths associated with dieting programs.

One of highest risks for sudden death syndrome in weight loss is during very low calorie diets, warn researchers at the NIH Obesity Research Center in New York. Fatal cardiac arrhythmias with these large, rapid losses may be related to reduced heart size.

The Federal Trade Commission charged six VLCD companies with false and misleading statements about both the safety and effectiveness of their programs in the three years following the 1990 congressional hearings. These six programs and their companies charged are: Optifast, Sandoz Nutrition; Ultrafast, National Center for Nutrition of Virginia; Medifast, Jason Pharmaceuticals and the Nutrition Institute of Maryland; HMR Fasting Program, Health Management Resources; UWCC Permanence Program and the Risk Reduction Program, United Weight Control Corporation; and New Directions, Abbott Laboratories. FTC said company advertising statements including, "Clinically proven safe," and "Without one instance of serious side effects associated with their treatment," are unsubstantiated.[4]

Minnesota starvation study

The classic starvation study is the Minnesota Experiment. A wartime effort in 1944-1945 involving 32 male volunteers, the purpose of the study was to find ways to improve life in war-torn countries after the war. The outcomes of this study provide important information on the adverse effects of rapid weight loss, and are detailed in an impressive two-volume work, *The Biology of Human Starvation* by Ancel Keys.

The study lasted one year: three months of an initial control period, six months of semi-starvation, and three months of re-feeding. Extensive testing was done at each stage and during the following year.

The diet fed to the men was intended to mimic the diet of starving people in occupied countries of Europe, such as Holland. Comprised mainly of vegetables, especially root vegetables, it was a diet high in carbohydrate, low in protein and with enough fat to make up the expected calories.

Averaging 1,570 calories, the diet was less than half the normal amount eaten by the men in the control period. The volunteers were required to lose 19 to 28 percent of body weight, depending on body composition (an average of 24 percent). If weekly weight loss for an individual fell short of what was expected, bread and potatoes were decreased; if weight loss was too high, these foods were increased.

Physical activity was vigorous. Each week the men walked 22 miles, participated in 30 minutes of treadmill testing, and worked 15 hours in clerical or maintenance work. They also walked a distance to the dining hall, adding another two to three miles each day. This level of physical activity was continued throughout the study, however researchers note that the quality of the men's work was poor during the final two months of semi-starvation.

As semi-starvation progressed, the men experienced profound physical and psychological changes. Many of these changes are also experienced by persons on weight loss diets.

As semi-starvation progressed, the men experienced profound physical and psychological changes.

Heart volume decreased 20 percent; metabolism fell almost 40 percent; all the men felt cold.

The following physical changes took place:

- Weight decreased an average of 24 percent, ranging from 18.8 to 29.3 percent (the men initially averaged 153 pounds, at 5-feet-10).

- Size decreased, especially in the diameter of upper thigh and upper arm where reduction was 25 percent; decrease in upper trunk breadth and depth, waist breadth and depth, pelvic depth, and neck breadth varied from about 9 to 15 percent.

- Heart volume decreased an average of about 20 percent; variability in heart volume was increased during starvation.

- Work output of heart per minute was reduced about 50 percent.

- Pulse rate slowed, from a mean of 56 initially to 37.8 beats per minute.

- Body temperature decreased slightly.

- Veins were less prominent, and often collapsed when blood was drawn.

- Basal metabolism rate fell by almost 40 percent by the end of 6 months of semi-starvation; metabolism was reduced per unit of tissue mass, as well as because of decreased size. This was calculated as equal to adaptive savings of 600 calories per day. (The researchers say some famine reports indicate women may have a greater decrease in metabolic rate than males, and also that women may have greater survival rates in times of starvation.)

- The men had an abnormal accumulation of fluid, which gave increased measurements for some in the ankle and wrist. (Edema is so closely related to semi-starvation that early terms linking the two were "hunger edema," "famine edema," and "war edema," writes Keys.)

- All the men felt cold and frequently complained of cold hands and feet. Even in mid-July, they wore jackets during the day and piled on blankets at night.

- The men felt weak and tired easily; voluntary movements became slower; their energy output decreased, even though regular physical activity was maintained including 20 miles of hiking per week.

- Their capacity to work decreased, especially that involving lifting, pushing and carrying loads. Also diminished was their ability to climb, walk long distances, and stand for long periods. Speed and accuracy were less impaired.

- Forearm, legs and back strength decreased by about 30 percent.

- Decrease in endurance.

- Giddiness and momentary blackouts upon rising were common.

- Frequent reports of muscle cramp, soreness, and extremities that "went to sleep"; tendon reflexes were more sluggish.

- Frequency of urination.

- No increase in diarrhea, bloating, flatulence or colic such as has been observed in natural starvation areas.

- Sexual function and testes size was reduced. (European famine reports frequently mention amenorrhea in women, impotence in men, delayed puberty in children, and decreased birth rate.)

- No impairment of visual ability was found, but there was an inability to focus, frequent eye-aches and spots before the eyes.

- Acuteness of hearing improved significantly, along with sensations of ringing in the head. Ordinary sounds were disturbing.

- Skin became pale, cold, dry, thin, scaly, rough, inelastic and marked with brownish pigmentation; skin ulcers and sores were common.

- Teeth and bones were apparently not demineralized as had been theorized; teeth were X-rayed at beginning and end, and decay was considered normal for a 6-month period. It is noted there is no evidence of teeth or bone deterioration from famine areas, and starving prisoners emerged from Japanese internment camps with teeth in remarkably good condition.

- Hair became thin, dry, and fell out.

- Senses of taste, smell and pressure seemed unaffected.

- The men appeared as if older, and behaved much older. They often said they felt old, but there were no indications of an accelerated aging process.

Effects in refeeding

- Physical discomforts continued after the restrictive diet ended, and the expected relief did not come quickly.

- The men gained fat tissue rapidly, and "soft roundness" became their dominant characteristic; in three months they had gained back an average of half their fat loss.

- Lean tissue recovered more slowly. Abdominal circumference reached 101 percent in three months for the highest calorie group, while arm, calf and thigh circumference recovered only 50 percent of initial size.

- The most rapid recovery was from dizziness, apathy and lethargy, with slower recovery from tiredness, weakness and loss of sex drive.

- Work capacity increased by week 13.

- The men had some problems with constipation, stomach pains, heartburn and gas, especially when they overate.

- Sleepiness and headaches increased for some.

- Thirst increased and edema continued to be a problem.[5]

(See Chapter 8 for psychological risks from the Minn. Study.)

Fad diets

The major medical risks for fad or gimmick diets are semi-starvation, nutrient deficiencies, and toxic reactions to unregulated "natural" or "herbal" supplements frequently advocated by health food promoters.

Fad diets often consist of specific food combinations such as steak

500 clients sue Nutri/System

Eighteen people from New York on Sept. 10 sued Nutri/System, Inc. of Blue Bell, Pa., for damage to their gallbladders, which had to be removed. They join more than 500 persons across the U.S. with similar lawsuits against the company. The first suits were filed in Florida 18 months ago. Five are scheduled to go to trial next month.

The recent suits allege that Nutri/System offers rapid weight loss, which may cause cholesterol-saturated bile to collect in the gallbladder and result in gallstones, according to Burt Bauman, the attorney representing the New York cases.

"The company didn't warn people that it was innately dangerous to lose rapidly like that. They had no medical supervision and people were losing three and four percent of their body weight a week," Bauman said. *(AP 9/11/91)*[52]

and grapefruit, or brown rice and tea, or all pineapple one day and all another food the next day. These "miracle" diets often leave out whole groups of foods which are essential in balanced, healthy eating.

Examples are the Rice Diet, the Water Diet, Dr. Atkins' Diet Revolution, Dr. Cooper's Fabulous Fructose Diet, the Scarsdale Medical Diet, the Mayo Clinic Diet (which is not a program of the Mayo Clinic), the Beverly Hills Diet, and Fit for Life.

Going vegetarian

Many women today have turned to vegetarianism in their fear of fat and for what they perceive as health reasons. They fear eating meat, even lean meat, because in the past it was often prepared with high-fat methods. Not only is this a futile effort – research shows American women are more likely to get their fat from baked goods and desserts than from meat – but it can lead to nutrition deficiencies, fatigue, apathy and irritabiity.

Certainly vegetarian diets can be healthy and well-balanced. But they must be carefully managed to provide the essential nutrition that is so easily available when even a small amount meat is included in the daily diet – and so often lacking when it is not. Protein from meat is complete and considered high-quality, while vegetable proteins may be incomplete and of lower quality. The heme iron in meat allows the mineral from plant sources to be easily absorbed in the body. Without meat, this iron may not be as available.

Anemia is extremely common among women and children in third world countries. This is a great loss in human potential and may account in part for an apathy toward bettering their conditions.

In the United States, 35 to 58 percent of young, healthy women have been found to have some degree of iron deficiency. In her child-bearing years, a woman's blood supply is depleted monthly through menstrual bleeding. During pregnancy, much blood is needed for the fetus and placenta; more blood is lost in delivery, and iron is needed in the milk supply. These losses can be severe for women.

Because they lack iron, so easily available from meat, many women all over the world are anemic, weak, passive, apathetic, self absorbed, irritable, depressed and submissive. Symptoms of iron deficiency include fatigue, decreased work capacity, pallor, palpitation and susceptibility to infection. The heart may become dilated and "hemic" murmurs heard. Often the person has cold hands and feet and vague stomach complaints, such as diarrhea, gas, nausea and constipation. Iron deficiency can contribute to underachievement and behavioral disturbances in children, growth retardation, and deficiency of thyroid hormone.[6]

Iron-deficient women have poorer control over their body temperature than other women, a Pennsylvania study shows. When cold-stressed, instead of generating more body heat and burning more calories to keep warm, their body temperature dropped 0.3 degrees C or more.[7] Other research found an iron-rich diet that included meat restored body temperature control. Real foods were found to be much more effective than iron supplements.[8]

Eating a balanced diet that includes meat may also help women to maintain normal eating patterns, and to avoid both overeating and disordered eating. A Swedish study found that women who ate a lunchtime casserole that included meat were satisfied longer, rated their meal higher

Chinese puzzle

An appalling example of the kind of rigid, restrictive youth weight loss program which should be behind us, but is not, comes from an AP story out of China. Reporting on growing obesity problems in China, the news story told of a 10-day weight-loss camp for children, attended by 60 youngsters, ages 8 to 14, directed by Dr. Yan Chun, chief endocrinologist at Beijing Children's Hospital.

Yan restricted his young campers to an 800 to 1,000 calorie, high protein, low starch, no-sweets diet. He exercised them four to five hours per day, and medicated them with a "new appetite suppressant."

The program "seems to be working," the reporter concluded, because, "the children's main topic of conversation was how much fat they'd shed."

The image represents a painful Chinese puzzle: Can you find the eight things wrong with this picture? (AP 2/27/91)[5]

in taste and satisfaction, and ate 12 percent fewer calories at the evening meal, than did women who ate a similar vegetarian casserole.

Low calorie diets

Moderate and balanced low calorie reducing diets today probably do not normally pose a risk to physical health, provided the lost weight is kept off and weight cycling is avoided. However, a matter of much current debate is whether dieting increases psychological abnormalities – such as restrained eating, bingeing, eating disorders, and other mental and emotional disturbances.

Low calorie reducing diets today are about 1,000 to 1,200 calories for women and 1,200 to 1,500 for men. Today it is expected that a healthy low calorie diet – like any moderate, balanced, healthy eating plan – will be high in carbohydrate, moderate in protein and low in fat. National dietary goals are for about 15 percent of total calorie intake to come from protein, 30 percent or less from fat, and 55 percent from carbohydrates, primarily starches. This is similar in protein, lower in fat, and higher in carbohydrate than the current average American diet. (Note that any calories consumed in alcohol must be added to make 100 percent, thus reducing the percent of other nutrients.)

In a balanced reducing diet, all five major food groups in a variety of foods will be included, as given in the USDA Food Pyramid. Eating a variety of these foods will insure getting the more than 50 nutrients needed by the body, in their best and most useable form.

A multivitamin that provides 100 percent or less of vitamins and mineral may be suggested by the dietitian along with a reducing diet. Megadose supplements may be toxic and are not recommended. Nutrition and health experts agree that it is far healthier to obtain nutrients from real foods than to rely on megadose supplements to improve a poor diet.

Because they lack iron, easily available in meat, many women all over the world are anemic, weak, passive, apathetic, self absorbed, irritable, depressed and submissive.

3. Diet pills and drugs

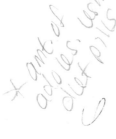

Widely available, diet pills are the weight loss drug of choice among teenagers.

Nearly 7 percent of adolescent girls in the U.S. are using diet pills, but many more have used them, according to the Center of Disease Control Youth Risk Behavior Surveillance System[1] Among adolescents who believe they are overweight, 34 percent have used diet pills to reduce weight. Of those trying to lose weight, 11 percent of girls and 3 percent of boys report using diet pills or diet candies within the past year.

In a study of 1,269 Cleveland high school students, 23 percent of the white girls and 16 percent of black girls had used diet pills. Only 6 percent of white boys and no black boys reported using diet pills.[2]

Diet pill abuse

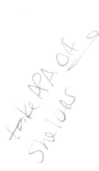

Diet pills with PPA (phenylpropanolamine), the nonprescription drug most commonly used in weight loss pills, are readily available in groceries, drug, chain and convenience stores. PPA and benzocaine are the only two drugs previously approved by FDA for nonprescription sales. This means drug claims can be made, about appetite suppressant effects. However, the efficacy and safety of both drugs is often questioned.

Abuse by both adults and children is widespread.

In a 1990 congressional hearing, committee members heard numerous pleas to take diet pills containing PPA off the shelves and restrict them to prescription, or to adults through pharmacy departments of drug stores.

Approved as a diet aid in 1979, PPA is found in such products as Dexatrim, Accutrim, Control, Dex-A-Diet, Diadex, Prolamine, Propagest, Rhinecon and Unitrol, and in some cold medicines. More than $40 million dollars are spent annually on advertising PPA diet products, says a subcommittee memo. Its sales go virtually unregulated.

Sales of PPA should be restricted for minors, said Vivian Meehan, president of the National Association of Anorexia Nervosa and Associated Disorders. She urged that diet pills, laxatives, diuretics and emetics be sold only under a doctor's prescription for those under age 18, and sold to adults from behind the pharmacy counter; never from an open shelf or near products identified as diet aids.

In a study of 1,368 female and 1,062 male students at Michigan State University, L. R. Krupka, professor of natural science, reported that nearly half the women and 6 percent of the men had taken a PPA dietary drug; 27 percent of the women within the past 12 months; 3 percent in the past 24 hours.

Although most women didn't start using them until age 16, 19 percent began taking PPA diet pills much earlier, some as young as 12. Even 9 percent of those who perceived themselves as slightly underweight had used PPA diet pills in the last 12 months.

None had ever consulted a physician about their use, even though labels advise this for users under age 18.

Many took more than the recommended daily limit of 75 mg of PPA. About one-fourth of the women using diet pills had also double-

Ephedrine strikes again

The death of a Saratoga, Wisconsin woman has been attributed to cardiac arrythmia, or a coronary, brought on by ephedrine, a weight-losing drug commonly found in over-the-counter diet pills, according to the toxicology report. Wood County Coroner Bill Voight declared accidental the death of Pamela Bradley, 30, found dead at her home Nov. 18, 1993.[51]

dosed, using other over-the counter, PPA-containing products at the same time. One woman with a severe cold had taken a diet pill and four non-prescription decongestant products containing PPA within 24 hours of the interview – a total of 675 mg.

Daily use of appetite suppressant diet pills may cause a rebound effect of fatigue and hyperphagia, insomnia, mood changes, irritability and, in extremely large doses, psychosis, say Allan Kaplan and Paul Garfinkel in *Medical issues and the Eating Disorders.*[3]

Questionable products

A great many fraudulent weight loss products are on the market which make drug claims outright or suggest them. They evade regulation by claiming to be food supplements, not drugs.

Of over-the-counter or nonprescription drugs, currently only PPA and benzocaine are allowed to make drug claims for weight loss. Drug claims are claims that the product can alter body functions such as suppressing appetite, speeding up metabolism, reducing fat, or blocking out calories, fat or sugar.

In some cases these are harmless. But every year deaths are reported from products like CalBan 3000. Another example is ephedrine, which is sold legally as a stimulant. But often it is marketed with names that imply weight loss, such as MiniSlim.

In March 1994, 10 Texas teenagers were taken to emergency rooms after overdosing on ephedrine. The stimulant was also suspected in the April 1994 heart attack death of a 43-year-old Austin woman. Friends said the woman was taking diet pills. In excess, ephedrine can cause a heart attack, stroke or seizures, the Dallas Morning News reported.[4] The death of a 30-year-old Saratoga, Wisc., woman was attributed to a coronary brought on by ephedrine in a weight loss product, according to the toxicology report.[5]

Weight loss quackery today relies heavily on the exploitation of herbs and "natural" products. This works because Congress has allowed herbal products to be sold as foods, as long as no drug claims are made on the label. Illegal drug claims are often made in advertising and literature.

An army of questionable vitamin and supplement dealers today is working to convince the American public that taking multi pills in multidoses will make up for supposed deficiencies and toxicities in our food supply. Never mind that our food supply in the U.S. is the safest and most wholesome it has ever been, equal to the best in the world.

It's apparent that there is more fraudulent and misleading information about nutrition today than there has ever been, and it is marketed effectively, with enormous profits, in high-tech, highly targeted ways.

Scam artists imply that because herbs are natural they are safe. This is not necessarily true. Many are actually toxic. Furthermore, raw, crude herbs can vary greatly in strength, since there is no regulation or standard dosages. The FDA says many cases of illness have been reported from herbal products, many of which contain potent drugs, and some people have died. However, the agency takes action against herbals only on a case-by-case basis, and usually only after injury complaints.

In 1985 the Food and Drug Administration documented more than 100 cases of adverse reactions to Herbalife weight loss products, includ-

In a college study nearly half the women had taken a PPA diet pill, 19 percent before age 16 – some began as young as 12.

ing nausea, headaches, diarrhea, constipation and vomiting and investigated several fatalities. Ingredients like mandrake and pokeroot, which posed a potential danger in some Herbalife products are no longer being used, says the company. Bee pollen has caused fatal allergic reactions. The FDA warns that although promoters claim it is "naturally safe" and "safe for any dieter," bee pollen is hazardous for persons with allergies, asthma or hay fever.[6]

Authorities in Australia linked royal bee jelly to a severe asthma attack that killed an 11-year-old girl.[7]

The weight loss product "Quickly" was recently found by FDA to contain the prescription drug furosemide in amounts that could be dangerous. Excessive doses can lead to profound depletion of water and electrolytes, blood volume reduction, dangerously low blood pressure, heart complications, nausea, diarrhea, vomiting, hearing loss, dizziness, headache and rash, said FDA.[8]

Health fraud works because people want to believe there are simple cures and easy ways to alter their imperfections. The quack exploits this with a mixture of mysticism, pseudoscience and sensationalism, says Burton Love, FDA Midwest Regional Director.

In 1994 the FDA introduced the MedWatch program for speeding up health care provider reporting of adverse reactions such as to nonprescription diet pills. The problem has been that there is an effective reporting system for prescription drugs but not for over-the-counter drugs. (MedWatch, FDA, 5600 Fishers Lane, Rockville, MD 20852-9787).

Smoking has its own powerful industry effectively promoting nicotine as a method of weight control.

Smoking

Tobacco use is responsible for more than one of every six deaths in the U.S., according to the Public Health Service Healthy People 2000. It is the most important single preventable cause of death and disease in this country. Cigarette smoking accounts for about 390,000 deaths yearly including 21 percent of all coronary heart disease deaths, 87 percent of lung cancer deaths, and 30 percent of all cancer deaths. Smoking during pregnancy accounts for 20 to 30 percent of low birth weight babies, up to 14 percent of preterm deliveries, and about 10 percent of all infant deaths.

While there is a decline in smoking, the decline has been slower among women than men.[9]

Smoking delivers what is probably the most commonly used – and dangerous – weight control drug of all: nicotine. Smoking has its own powerful industry effectively promoting nicotine as a method of weight control.

One study of students, faculty and staff at a large southern university found 39 percent of female smokers and 25 percent of male smokers were using smoking to avoid weight gain. Twenty percent of overweight women smokers had started smoking to control their weight. Of those who had tried to quit, subsequent weight gain and increased appetite were major reasons for their return to smoking.[10]

Nicotine increases metabolism, according to a Swiss study which found smoking 24 cigarettes a day increases calorie expenditure by 10 percent. Average heart rate increased 20 percent with smoking.

Numerous studies confirm the popular belief that smoking helps keep weight down. A great deal of evidence shows that smokers tend to

Dieters light up more often

People on weight loss programs may be more likely to increase their smoking, according to a Brown University study. The researchers tested the nicotine intake, through analyzing codinine in the saliva, of 18 women smokers on a 26-week program which included 12 weeks on a very low calorie diet program. The 9 women completing the program lost an average 54 pounds, while steadily increasing their concentration of codinine, suggesting higher rates of smoking.

It is speculated that increase in smoking may be due to increased anxiety, a desire to suppress appetite or increase energy expenditure.[52]

weigh less and that, for many people, quitting smoking promotes weight gain.[11]

However, it has also been shown that for both men and women the weight gain with quitting smoking brought them only up to the average weight of persons who had never smoked. Average gain with quitting smoking was six pounds for men and eight pounds for women in this study.[12]

Thus, nicotine acts much like prescription anorectic drugs. Drugs may help the patient lose about ten pounds, it is reported; this is usually kept off while the drug is being taken, then is regained when the patient goes off the drug.

Dangerous responses

Paul Raford, MD, technical advisor to the congressional subcommittee conducting the hearings, testified that even when used correctly, PPA can cause dangerous reactions. It leads all other major non-prescription drugs in the number of adverse drug reactions and in number of contacts with Poison Control Centers, nearly 47,000 in 1989, he said.

The subcommittee found documented cases of fatal strokes, dangerously high blood pressure, heart rhythm abnormalities, heart muscle and kidney damage, hallucinations, seizures, psychosis, headaches, nervousness and insomnia from PPA use.

Other risks of PPA given in testimony by Denise Bruner, MD, Alexandria, VA, are cerebral hemorrhage, increased intercerebral pressure, nausea, vomiting, anxiety, palpitations, reversible renal failure, disorientation, psychotic behavior and death.

Further, said Raford, PPA is regarded by most users as ineffective, and he says no data at all contradicts this.

Exaggerated claims

Thaddeus Prout, MD, former chairman of the FDA Committee on Anorectic Drugs, questioned both the effectiveness and safety of PPA. He recalled being a part of the "chaotic and irresponsible decision-making process" under which PPA was reviewed.

"In July of 1983 we discussed this same question with all of the sophistication of academia going up against the billions of dollars of profits of the rapacious drug industry. We listened to their data, looked at their paltry studies.

"When the smoke cleared in July 1983, and the bombast was silent, we carried off our wounded, some of whom were able to settle out of court for the various misfortunes that had befallen them. Gloria Davis, a quadriplegic at age 26 was awarded $125 million for a lifetime disability.

"(Now) we are hearing all the exaggerated claims of success again. The same faces, the same people who have been doing industry-paid research for two decades are before us.

"Unfortunately it is very hard to prove that the disasters caused by this industry are grossly under-reported. One cannot treat obesity with 12 weeks of pill therapy. One cannot allow patients to take dangerous drugs without supervision."

Prout accused the industry of trying to dismiss death and injury as mere anecdotes. "We need to say a word about anecdotes. The thalido-

"We are hearing all the exaggerated claims of success again. The same people who have been doing industry-paid research for two decades. We listened to their data, looked at their paltry studies."

mide debacle started as a series of unconfirmed and unstudied anecdotes. Cerebral vascular hemorrhages, many fatal in women on birth control pills, were anecdotal. Tampons as a cause of Toxic Shock Syndrome was unconfirmed for years . . .

"And so it goes, with one difference. An aroused FDA acted promptly at those times.

"The purpose of reporting adverse reactions has always been to define a problem and do something constructive about it. (But) the medical profession has learned they need not waste the time (with) an entrenched and persuasive pharmaceutical industry. A suggestion eight years ago to consider making these medications prescription drugs was considered unworkable, without even looking at the possibility.

"Shall we wait another decade and have a new generation of concerned physicians wringing their hands and bumping their heads against the stone wall of industry?"

Wyden charged that most studies supporting PPA are seriously flawed. "Since the mid-1960s, the Food and Drug Administration has been involved in a running battle with the medical profession regarding the FDA's conclusion that PPA is both safe and effective as an over-the-counter drug. Goaded by concerned physicians, the FDA is once again reviewing PPA. Meanwhile, sales of PPA products soar, and the consumer protection efforts of other agencies are stymied."

Wyden also charged FDA and other federal regulatory agencies with being "sleeping watchdogs," and abandoning many of their enforcement responsibilities through the 1980s. Nearly 20 years had lapsed, he said, since the FDA began drafting regulations to ban more than a hundred other unsafe and ineffective ingredients used in diet pills.

Stung by Wyden's accusations, the FDA acted to ban 111 ingredients previously used in fraudulent and questionable diet pills. The much-delayed investigation began before 1975, and became effective as a ban Feb. 10, 1992.[13]

Guar gum was declared a hazard by FDA in this action, bringing to an end the long-extended Cal-Ban 3000 debacle in which at least one person died and more than 50 were injured, mostly due to throat obstruction.

This occurred five years after the U.S. Postal Service barred Cal-Ban 3000 from the mails, in 1987. Other federal regulatory agencies delayed while Cal-Ban's blatantly false and misleading advertisements flooded the airwaves and the consumer press. On the strength of its aggressive advertising, and enormous profitability, Cal-Ban entered mainstream markets through chain drug stores and discount outlets and enjoyed heavy sales.[14]

Stung by Wyden's accusations, the FDA banned 111 ingredients used in fraudulent and questionable diet pills.

4. Purging, exercise

Numerous other potentially hazardous weight loss methods are in use today by children as well as adults. They include vomiting, abuse of laxatives, diuretics and ipecac syrup, enemas, dehydration, dangerous gadgetry, withholding needed medication, and even obsessive exercise.

Vomiting

Self-induced vomiting is a purging behavior practiced by some youngsters and adults in trying to control their weight. It can cause many medical complications.

In a study of Cleveland high school students, 16 percent of white girls, 3 percent of black girls, and 7 percent of white boys had used vomiting to lose weight. No black male students had used this method, although their dieting rates were about the same as for white males (41-42%). Eight percent of all white girls vomited monthly or more often to lose weight.[1]

Among those adolescents who see themselves as overweight 23 percent have used vomiting to reduce weight. One-third of female high school students and 15 percent of male students say they are overweight, in the Center of Disease Control Youth Risk Behavior Surveillance, even though the actual rate is about 21 percent. Of the girls, 44 percent are currently trying to lose weight including 27 percent of those who think they're about the right weight, says this report.[2]

"Harmful weight loss practices and negative attitudes about body size have been reported among girls as young as nine years of age," CDC warns.

Those who vomit to control weight commonly complain of a heartburn-type pain from the gastric acid's irritating effect on the esophageal lining, say Philip Mehler and Kenneth Weiner, eating disorder specialists.[3]

Upper gastrointestinal tract irritation may result in sore throats, difficulty in swallowing and indigestion. Forceful vomiting may also cause small tears in the mucosa of the gastrointestinal tract with blood in the vomitus. Occasionally, the force of vomiting may cause breaking of small blood vessels in the eyes. It may cause injury to the esophageal sphincter to allow stomach contents into the lower esophagus.

The esophagus can rupture after ingestion of a large meal and subsequent forceful vomiting. This is a medical emergency with very severe upper abdominal pain, worsened by swallowing and breathing. It has a high mortality rate if left untreated and surgery is usually needed.

Prolonged vomiting may cause loss of potassium, an electrolyte, essential for muscle and heart functioning. Low levels can trigger cardiac arrhythmias.

Induced vomiting can cause so-called "chipmunk" cheeks, probably due to repeated stimulation of these glands by the acid contents of the stomach. These swollen facial glands usually go down with cessation of vomiting, but in some cases they may be difficult to reduce and can cause a worsening of the person's cosmetic self-image.

Persons who induce vomiting three times a week or more will eventually show erosion of tooth enamel from the frequent presence of acid

Among adolescents who see themselves as overweight 23 percent have used vomiting to reduce weight.

Ipecac syrup is extremely dangerous. It can cause cardiovascular, gastrointestinal and neuromuscular toxicity.

vomitus in the mouth, say Mehler and Weincr. This has been reported after only six months, but can take several years. This effect can cause sensitivity to heat or cold, spaces between the teeth, loss of fillings and general deterioration of the teeth.

R. John McComb, associate professor of Oral Pathology University of Toronto, says dentists need to be aware of excessive tooth erosion due to vomiting. Patients with eating disorders may come to them because of pain but try to hide the cause.

Tooth damage comes in three stages, he explains. First is erosion of enamel. Second is erosion and attrition of enamel and dentin. Third is loss of vertical tooth height. As enamel erodes, teeth appear unnaturally smooth and dull with a change to yellowness from the underlying dentin. Eventually the enamel is perforated and the dentin exposed, a stage that may typically take about seven years. Later the pulp may be exposed, usually with much pain. Height is reduced as teeth become thinner and sharper; edges break off and wear away more quickly, reducing the tooth to half or one third its original height. In molars, a crater developing in the center causes thinner edges which then begin wearing down. Grinding of the teeth due to anxiety may increase tooth wear.

Although most dentists are not trained in consulting bulimic patients, it is important to know facial and other symptoms, find what is occurring, establish trust, and persuade the patient to seek further treatment, a process which may take months, McComb suggests.[4]

Ipecac syrup may be used to induce vomiting. This contains the alkaloid emetine for promoting vomiting. However, the body develops a tolerance, so the user ingests increasingly larger doses. It is extremely dangerous and can cause cardiovascular, gastrointestinal and neuromuscular toxicity.[5]

Cuts and callouses on the hands or fingers from inducing the gag reflex may be noticable symptoms of vomiting behavior.

Laxatives and diuretics

The Cleveland high school study that looked at diet pill use among teens also studied use of laxatives and diuretics. The findings:[6]

	Laxatives	Diuretics
	Percent using	
Black girls	18%	11%
White girls	7	5
White boys	5	1
Black boys	2	2

Laxatives are an ineffective and dangerous method of weight loss. Superficially, they cause weight loss through chronic dehydration due to a large volume of watery diarrhea, explain University of Colorado eating disorder specialists Philip Mehler and Kenneth Weiner. Calorie absorption is not really affected. However, nutrients such as protein and calcium may be poorly absorbed.[7]

Laxative abuse can cause both acute and chronic lower gastrointestinal complications, including abdominal cramping, bloating, pain, nausea, constipation and diarrhea, say eating disorder specialists Amy Baker Dennis, PhD, and Randy Sansone, MD, in their "Overview of eating disorders," written for the National Eating Disorders Organization.[8]

They say that laxative abuse may also cause malabsorption of fat, protein and calcium. Laxatives can result in the loss of electrolytes, including potassium, which is essential for heart function. As potassium level drops, the likelihood of heart arrhythmias increases.

Chronic abuse may cause nerve damage resulting in sluggish bowel function. This happens as the colon becomes thin, dilated and lacking in normal propulsive action. This can become so severe that removal of the colon is needed in advanced cases, to be replaced by a colectomy.

Tolerance develops over time to laxatives and instead of the usual dose of one or two tablets only, individuals often take up to 60 or more tablets daily. Laxatives are probably the most common type of drug abused by bulimic patients, eating disorder specialists say.[9]

Diuretics or water pills are used less often by youngsters, but this abuse is extremely dangerous. The big concern here is potassium loss in heart arrhythmia as well as kidney damage. Diuretic abuse can cause rapid and dramatic potassium loss and dehydration.

Using several purging techniques together can intensify the overall effects on potassium and fluid loss. A physician should be consulted immediately with signs of potassium loss such as muscle weakness, fatigue and chest pain, according to Dennis and Sansone.

Gadgetry, wraps

Various weight loss gadgets may also pose health risks and have caused harm to users. The promoters of Gut Buster, an exercise device, were recently charged by the Federal Trade Commission with failing to disclose that the spring-tension device might break and injure the user. They were also charged with false and misleading advertising about Gut Buster's effectiveness for toning and trimming the stomach.[10]

Plastic wraps, the wearing of plastic garments while exercising, or excessive time spent in hot saunas to increase weight loss may contribute to dehydration and heat stroke.

The study found 36 percent of the women were withholding insulin for weight control.

Withholding medications

Some necessary medications may inadvertently promote weight gain. This can cause a deep concern for some individuals. They may refuse to take their medications, or avoid taking them regularly, despite suffering severe or noticable ill effects.

A psychiatric study at the University of Texas investigated the extent of withholding insulin among a group of 42 women, age 16 to 40, with insulin-dependent diabetes (IDDM). The study found 15 of the women, or 36 percent, were insulin withholders. These women were withholding insulin for weight control, placing themselves at risk for severe hyperglycemia, diabetic ketoacidosis, and increased risk of long-term complications of diabetes.

The study found insulin withholders were more concerned with dieting and weight gain, were more likely to binge eat, and reported more body image disturbance problems than women who did not withhold insulin. They were more likely to have dysfunctional self-perceptions, inadequacy and alienation feelings, negative attitudes toward diabetes, a reluctance to develop close relationships and to describe their social relationships as tense and disappointing.[11]

Obsessive exercise

In increasing numbers men and women are seeking counseling for compulsive exercise – usually not because they want to stop, but because they are unable to continue, according to Karin Kratina, MA, RD, a dietitian, exercise physiologist and clinical outreach coordinator at the Renfrew Center in Florida.[12]

Kratina describes a typical young woman with exercise dependence. She rises each morning at 5:30, hits the pavement for a brisk three miles, rain or shine, works out 45 minutes at the fitness center on lunch break, and goes to another health club after work for an hour of aerobics, half an hour on the Stairmaster and a half hour on the Lifecycle. She appears to be a motivated, fit and happy person but her legs ache constantly, as she continues to work out despite shin splints. When she stops for a time her depression and anxiety become so overwhelming, she can't wait to get back to her workouts.

Excessive exercise aimed at weight loss is regarded as a secondary dependency, usually to an eating disorder. Pure exercise dependence is found most often in middle-aged men in their 40's and 50's, says Kratina. In this case, weight loss is seen as a means to improve performance, and typically weight is not allowed to drop too low.

As many as 7 percent of committed exercisers may be dependent on exercise to the point it interferes with their lives. Kratina suggests that at least half of anorexics and bulimics probably deal with some form of exercise dependency.

Physical activity takes priority over everything else for the exercise dependent individual. He or she follows stereotyped patterns, continues exercising even when a serious physical disorder is known to be caused or aggravated by it, and experiences severe withdrawal symptoms upon being forced to stop for a time.

"Stress injuries are common, and frequently the person exercises right through an injury so it can't heal properly," says Kratina.

Risks with normal exercise

A moderate exercise program which progresses gradually is generally safe and highly recommended for nearly everyone. It is especially important in weight management programs.

However, exercise can constitute a risk which should not be ignored. Even a reasonable program can involve risks for certain individuals, or others under certain conditions.

The Michigan Health Council recommends that people in weight management programs be screened for conditions which could make exercise hazardous for them, and be monitored for abnormal responses during exercise. The Michigan report, *Toward Safe Weight Loss,* includes the following precautions.[13]

Reasons for medical clearance before exercise

- History of heart disease, stroke, chest pain diagnosed as angina pectoris, known cardiac dysrhythmias or conduction defects.
- Use of medications for the heart or blood vessels during the last three months.
- Any acute infectious disease.

As many as 7 percent of committed exercisers may be dependent on exercise to the point it interferes with their lives.

- Neuromuscular, musculoskeletal or orthopedic disorders that would make walking uncomfortable or dangerous.
- Renal (kidney), hepatic (liver) or other metabolic problems.
- Resting blood pressure greater than 160 mmHg systolic or 100 mmHg diastolic.
- Previous medical advice not to exercise.
- Any suspicion that exercise may be harmful.

Symptoms of abnormal response

Stop exercising and see your physician before resuming your training program if any of the following occur:

1. Chest pain or pressure, pain in the arm, throat, or jaw during or immediately after exercise.
2. Dizziness, lightheadedness, confusion, sudden lack of coordination, cold sweating, glassy stare, nausea, or fainting.
3. Abnormal heart activity such as many noticeable extra beats, fluttering, palpitations in the chest or throat, or sudden bursts of rapid heart beats.

If any of the above symptoms persist, seek emergency care.

Drink enough fluids to prevent dehydration and overheating.

Exercise is a priority

The Michigan guidelines recommend that people engage in 30 to 60 minutes of continuous physical activity five to seven times per week, preferably in low impact activities such as walking, cycling and swimming which are less likely to cause injury. The activity should be consistent with individual interests so it can be maintained indefinitely.

Weight loss programs should include an exercise component which is safe and appropriate to the individual. It is clear that exercise can increase long term success, increase energy expenditure, help maintain lean body mass, improve functional capacity, reduce cardiovascular risk and promote a sense of personal well-being.

5. Surgery

Weight-reduction surgery may be advocated for patients with obesity-related risk factors or lifestyle limitations. This surgery should, in general, be reserved for patients who are at least 100 pounds over their so-called "desirable" weight, or who have a body mass index greater than 40, according to recommendations.

About 15,000 weight-reduction surgeries are performed in the U.S. annually, according to Thomas Blommers, Executive Manager of the American Society for Bariatric Surgery.

Costs vary according to areas of the country and type of procedure, but often range from $25,000 to $30,000 for the surgery, pre-operative testing, and hospital stay of five or six days. This does not include follow-up complications or reoperative procedures. Most surgeries are paid by insurance, says Blommers.

The Food and Nutrition Board of the Institute of Medicine published a 1995 report "Weighing the Options: Criteria for evaluating weight-management programs" in which members of the board seem to advocate a wider use of weight-reduction surgery.

"It is puzzling that this treatment (gastric surgery) is not more widely used for severely obese individuals at very high risk for obesity-related morbidity and mortality. It is possible that health care providers and individuals alike fail to fully understand the severity and costs of obesity in terms of both increased morbidity and mortality and its impact on the quality of life. Perhaps there is also an intrinsic fear of the dangers of surgery due in part to lack of knowledge. In fact, mortality associated with gastric surgery for obesity is less than 1 percent," said the report.[1]

Improvement in related risk factors and lifestyle often follow this surgery and its accompanying weight loss.

Yet the operation carries a high risk of complications and death. For elective surgery the death of one patient in every hundred is, after all, not an inconsiderable risk. Also it is generally accepted that some or much weight is commonly regained within two to five years.

> *The first two years after surgery are called the "honeymoon period" by size activists.*

Surgical risks

The first two years after surgery are called "the honeymoon period" by size acceptance activists. They call for an end to weight-reduction surgery because of the severe longterm complications many have suffered from this surgery.

A recent study in Norway supports findings that the first two years are the most favorable.

Five-year results may be very different than those after the first two or three years, the Norwegian researchers report. Many of their gastric banding surgery patients had late complications, and fewer than half maintained their weight within 30 percent of desirable for five years.

These surgeons performed 174 vertical banded gastroplasties between 1981 and 1985, choosing this procedure in preference to the previously used gastric bypass for its lower mortality and complication rate.

Twenty-five complications reported during the first 30 days included severe wound infections. Gastric perforation occurred in four patients. One was discovered early enough to make repairs and postpone the operation. Three developed peritonitis and were re-operated; two recovered and one died due to septicaemia and multi-organ failure. Five required intravenous infusion for more than one week for gastric retention. Another patient was re-operated because of wound dehiscence. Two had post-operative venous thrombosis and one had a small pulmonary embolism.

After five years, a total of 60 late complications were registered in 48 patients. Twenty-six patients were re-operated, 24 with removal of the band, 13 because of gastric retention with unacceptable vomiting. Incisional hernia occurred in 15 patients, of whom six were operated. There were a total of four deaths, one clearly unrelated, one unknown.

Rapid weight loss occurred the first six months, then leveled off to an average loss of 36.5 kg at 12 months. The number of patients who maintained their weight at or below the 30 percent of desirable was 69 percent at one year after surgery, 60 percent at two years, and 47 percent at five years. At one year only 9 percent weighed more than 50 percent over desirable, but by five years this had risen to 27 percent. The researchers note that many studies have shown acceptable weight loss and complication rates in two to three year follow-up, but that their five year results have changed "our early optimistic view to a more realistic one." They now suggest that gastric banding (probably the most frequently used operation today for weight reduction) is not a final solution to the problems of obesity.[2]

Figure 2

DATTA panel deadlocks on weight loss surgery

1. Is gastric bypass surgery (A) a safe and (B) an effective adjunctive therapy to diet, exercise and behavior modification programs in the treatment of resistant cases of morbid obesity?

	Established	Investigational	Unacceptable	Indeterminate
A. Safety	42%	40%	13%	5%
B. Effectiveness	45	42	10	3

2. Is vertical-banded gastroplasty (A) a safe and (B) an effective adjunctive therapy to diet, exercise and behavior modification programs in the treatment of resistant cases of morbid obesity?

	Established	Investigational	Unacceptable	Indeterminate
A. Safety	54%	38%	5%	3%
B. Effectiveness	46	41	5	8

Answers given as percent of DATTA panelists. Safety is defined as having a low risk of harm, injury or loss; effectiveness as producing a desired, beneficial effect under conditions of actual use. Definitions are: Established - demonstrated and accepted as safe and effective; Investigational - technology largely confined for use under research protocol; Unacceptable - an unfavorable risk/benefit ratio; Indeterminate - evidence is insufficient for a definitive decision.

Weight reduction surgery was evaluated for safety and effectiveness by a panel of 38 specialists in surgery and gastroenterology for the American Medical Association in 1989. Although this Diagnostic and Therapeutic Assessment (DATTA) panel studied reports in the scientific literature through 1988, panel members could not reach a consensus, and remained sharply divided on both issues and for both types of surgery. Morbidity is estimated at 10 percent and mortality at 1 percent for these gastric reduction surgeries, in the DATTA report.[2]

JAMA 1989/HEALTHY WEIGHT JOURNAL(O&H) 1991

"*The legacy of the NIH panel's endorsement of intestinal bypass surgery is perhaps a hundred thousand patients worldwide, the majority of whom have suffered severe complications.*"

– Paul Ernsberger

Paul Ernsberger, PhD, assistant professor of medicine at Case Western Reserve University School of Medicine in Cleveland, reports that the maximum benefit from lasting weight loss is a five-year prolonging of life for women, comparing the longevity of normal-weight women with those with a body mass index of 40 or more. Therefore any risks from treatment, such as surgery, must be kept low to justify these benefits. Further, even though it is recommended that the surgery be reserved for patients with severe obesity, many exceptions are made and there is a trend to operate on thinner patients, he reports.

One woman who had this surgery at a weight of 209 pounds because her movements were limited from polio, explained, "I made the decision that I would rather die on the operating table than to continue to gain weight as I had been doing, " she said.[3]

Potential benefits of weight-reduction surgery need to be carefully and openly weighed against its risks, so patients as well as physicans can make informed decisions. An acceptable mortality rate for this surgery has not been determined.

The DATTA panel of 38 experts convened by the American Medical Association in 1989 could not reach a consensus on whether to declare safe or effective either of the two most acceptable surgeries for weight reduction. After a thorough review, only 42 percent of the surgery and gastroenterology specialists agreed that the safety of gastric bypass surgery is established. Only 54 percent said safety is established for vertical-banded gastroplasty. The split on effectiveness was similar: 45 percent said the gastric bypass is effective and 46 percent called the gastroplasty effective. From the evidence presented, the DATTA panel estimated a death rate of 1 percent and morbidity of 10 percent for these surgeries.

Other higher risk surgeries, such as the biliopancreatic bypass and intestinal bypass, were not evaluated by the AMA panel.

When surgery is done at major surgery centers, a much lower mortality rate is reported, insists R. Armour Forse, MD, PhD, assistant professor of surgery at Harvard Medical School. In a review of 5,178 patients from 12 medical centers he says the overall mortality rate was only 0.008 percent. Forse compared this favorably to the mortality rate of 0.03 percent for morbidly obese men of the same age. He does not compare the rate for women, or give the length of the post-operative period studied, however.[4]

There is an inconsistancy in reporting surgical deaths. Some surgeons or researchers report only deaths during surgery or immediately postoperative. Others believe late deaths, including suicides, are very relevant to this type of surgery. This information is often lacking in reports.

A Canadian report in *Surgery 1990* [5] discussing three deaths in 201 patients, says one patient died of pulmonary embolism 30 days after surgery; another died of myocardial infarction 18 months after surgery, after losing 36 percent of initial weight; and the third, a 51-year-old woman, died of suicide 30 months after surgery.

In reporting late mortality from two studies with a total of 490 patients, Forse says one had four late deaths and none during the operation. The other had three late deaths and no operative deaths. Of these seven deaths, three were suicides; the others were due to "obesity related" problems.

The high suicide rate has not been explained.

Surgical accountability

A National Institutes of Health Consensus Conference on Gastrointestinal Surgery for Severe Obesity was held in 1991. The conference statement approved the two gastric surgeries but called for better statisitical reporting of surgical results, particularly long-term effects and survival.[6]

According to the conference report: Weight lost is generally greatest by 18 to 24 months after surgery, followed by some degree of regain. Lack of adequate studies make evaluation difficult, and quality of life considerations need to be addressed: "The euphoria seen commonly in patients in the early postoperative period may be supplanted later by significant depression."

Nutrient deficiencies are common after stomach reducing surgery. Iron deficiency anemia is a frequent longterm complication of gastric bypass surgery.

Ernsberger charges that there is a lack of sufficient prior animal testing for this type of surgery. Other surgical techniques are first developed in the animal laboratory, then run in controlled clinical trials which compare long-term outcomes with a control group. They are then refined with further animal studies. But with gastric surgery, he says, sufficient controlled trials are not conducted.

Surgeons are relatively free to perform their preferred types of surgery or a variation of approved surgeries. Not all confine their weight reduction surgeries to the generally approved types. Some prefer methods such as the biliopancreatic bypass because the resulting malabsorption of food makes weight reduction more effective, even though risk of severe complications may be greater. A surgeon may work independently, experimenting on individual patients with variations which differ widely in safety and effectiveness.

The earlier 1987 NIH conference on this weight-reduction surgery approved the intestinal bypass surgery at a time when that operation was under fire for its numerous adverse effects, and just before it was disavowed, Ernsberger said. But because of the endorsement from the NIH conference, the operation was accepted for health insurance coverage of tens of thousands of operations. Intestinal bypass is no longer recommended due to its severe complications.

"The legacy of the NIH panel's endorsement of intestinal bypass surgery is perhaps a hundred thousand patients worldwide, the majority of whom have suffered severe complications. Of the survivors, most now have had the operation undone," said Ernsberger.[7]

A typical patient for this type of surgery is a woman in her 30s, he reports. She faces another four decades of life, which means that to gain health benefits, her weight loss must be maintained for at least 10 years and preferably 20. He says her surgery risk must be low to make it worthwhile.

More definitive answers on the value and risks of surgery are expected to result from the ongoing SOS Swedish study (Swedish Obese Subjects). This is an ambitious 10-year study of obesity and its treatment which will include 2,000 gastric surgery patients along with 2,000 matched controls. By the end of 1994, this group included 500 patients and 500 controls who had been followed for two years. Currently, the researchers

The high suicide rate has not been explained.

say more patients and a longer follow up are needed to answer the questions of whether mortality and morbidity are decreased or increased after surgery.[8]

Support programs giving nutritional, medical and psychological counseling for obesity surgery are clearly needed, but not always provided, says the consensus statement.

Types of surgery

Of the two most common types of weight-reduction surgeries in the U.S., vertical banded gastroplasty is less complex and has fewer complications than Roux-enY gastric bypass, according to the 1995 "Weighing the Options," report of the National Academy of Sciences Institute of Medicine.[9] Gastric bypass is more effective in longterm weight loss, but has higher risk of perioperative complications and nutritional deficiencies. The report cites the development of gallstones in three-quarters of severely obese individuals who underwent gastric surgery in one study. Risks include postoperative complications, micronutrient deficiencies, "dumping syndrome," and late postoperative depression. Death rate in this 1995 report is given as "less than 1 percent," or fewer than one out of every 100 patients. The report says some of the weight loss is regained within two to five years.

The biliopancreatic diversion, long discouraged in the U.S. because of higher complication risk, is nevertheless being performed more today because of its greater weight loss. In addition to reducing food volume it causes malabsorption of food in bypassing part of the intestine.

The use of laparoscopic procedures is advancing quickly, says Blommers. But their relative simplicity may be deceptive. According to a statement of the American Society for Bariatric Surgery, "Laparoscopic obesity operations should be undertaken only by surgeons who are experienced in both laparoscopic and open bariatric techniques, and who understand the complexities of the surgical treatment of obesity."

Another type of widely promoted stomach intrusion was the Garren-Edwards gastric bubble which in 1985 received quick approval from FDA. Obesity specialists blame its hasty approval on publicity from the 1985 NIH conference which defined the health risks of obesity. Later the FDA reconsidered their approval, reduced the bubble to experimental basis, and finally withdrew it from the market. Independent controlled studies had proved it useless and revealed numerous adverse side effects.

Liposuction is a cosmetic or body shaping procedure to remove fat from certain areas of the body. Since only small amouts of fat are removed it should not be regarded as a weight loss procedure, although it may be promoted and viewed in this way. The most common risk from liposuction is severe bruising.

Complications can be overwhelming

A common complaint of weight-reduction surgery patients who suffer severe complications is that they were not told beforehand what can happen: months of hospitilization, foul odors, adverse food reactions, continual nausea, infection and abesses, pain from the staples, skin eruptions and exema, profound body changes, depression, nutrition deficiencies, severe diarrhea and the need to stay close to a bathroom. Then afterwards, they are "reassured" by numerous physicians that their

---

Liposuction ads

Minneapolis cosmetic surgeon Scott M. Ross has agreed to settle charges that he overpromised results and understated risks of liposuction in Minneapolis Center for Cosmetic Surgery advertisements. The Federal Trade Commission alleged that Ross falsely implied that liposuction, and the surgical removal of body fat by suction, is a low-risk procedure. Further, the FTC charged that "before" and "after" photographs in the ads misrepresented the typical results that can be achieved throug liposuction, and the amount of time it takes to achieve them.*(FTC 1992)*[51]

sometimes-permanently debilitating effects are common with this type of surgery.

They say they did not have the information they needed beforehand to make an informed decision. Had they known the possible complications, they might have been less eager to undergo major elective surgery, which they hoped would solve their problems, but instead added new ones.

When one considers that 15,000 or more surgeries are performed each year in the U.S. alone, with an expected 10 percent morbidity rate even from the two least intrusive methods, this suggests a great many patients are currently suffering severe complications.

A support group for these people, called "Weight Loss Surgery Survivors SIG," is sponsored by the National Association to Advance Fat Acceptance, and headquartered in Albuquerque, N.M. The group publishes a quarterly newsletter and provides information on surgery complications.

"I am appalled that doctors are convinced of the value of such surgery in advance of the data," said Karen Smith, coordinator of the group. "Surgeons are too busy operating to further investigate the safety and long-term effectiveness of weight loss surgery."[10]

William Fabrey, a founder of NAAFA, says, "Perhaps 10 percent of our members have had weight loss surgery at one time or another, have gained the weight back and suffered health problems as a result of the surgery. Unfortunately, two people I knew personally died after having this surgery."[11]

Weight loss surgery should be eliminated urges Miriam Berg, Woodstock, N.Y., president of the Council on Size and Weight Discrimination. "Life-threatening complications, chronic debilitation and severely diminished quality of life following such surgery should have ended this practice years ago, especially since a large percentage of patients regain all weight lost," said Berg.

Because of the severe adverse effects many of their members have suffered, both the Council and NAAFA call for an end to weight-reduction surgery.

"Life-threatening complications, chronic debilitation and severely diminished quality of life following such surgery should have ended this practice years ago."
— Miriam Berg

6. Sports and athletes

Athletes in sports and performance arts that emphasize leanness are at special risk for developing dangerous weight loss practices and eating disorders. For some of these athletes, losing weight becomes an all-consuming passion.

At special risk are top athletes in such sports as gymnastics, wrestling, judo, boxing, weight lifting, bodybuilding, figure skating, diving, ballet, dance, horse racing and distance running.

While anorexia nervosa may affect 0.4 to 1 percent of teenage girls in the general population, it has been found to affect as many as 13 to 22 percent of women in selected groups of elite runners and dancers.

Competing while dehydrated is extremely hazardous.

Struggling to be the best at a sport while coping with body changes in adolescence is especially difficult for girls, because of societal pressures that promote thinness and beauty. Trying to control weight while focusing on training and performance may lead to a sense of frustration, guilt, despair and failure – and to a pattern of unhealthy eating and eating disorders. Further, the athlete may share some of the traits of eating disorder patients in that they are driven, compulsive and goal oriented, according to Jacqueline Berning and Suzanne Steen, authors of *Sports Nutrition for the 90's.*[1]

Methods

The methods some of these athletes use to keep thin – rubber suits, exessive heat in saunas, diuretics, laxatives, self-induced vomiting, excessive exercise, semi-starvation and dehydration – have potentially dangerous consequences.

Weight control practices such as severely restricting food and fluid may affect metabolism, body composition, performance and overall health. Fluid losses and resulting electrolyte disturbances can increase risk of cardiac arrhythmias, renal damage, impaired performance and increased chance of injury, said David Garner and Lionel Rosen, eating disorder specialists, in the Journal of Applied Sport Science Research. These unorthodox weight control methods also can influence cardiac output and body temperature.[2]

Severe dieting affects both the mind and body. It is often reassuring for the athlete to know that symptoms he or she is experiencing – poor concentration, moodiness, irritability, anger, depression, feelings of inadequacy, anxiety, obsessional thinking, poor decision making and social withdrawal – may be consequences of dieting, and not necessarily signs of deeper emotional disturbances, say these researchers.

Dancers, skaters

In two studies of female dancers cited by Berning and Steen, between 5 and 22 percent had anorexia nervosa, with a higher incidence among adults than adolescents, and among women competing in national rather than regional performances.

A study that compared ballet dancers, figure skaters and swimmers with nonathletes found the dancers and skaters were lighter, leaner and more likely to have delayed menarche than the swimmers or nonathletes. They also had more eating disorder symptoms, with the dancers having the highest eating disorder scores of all.

Jockeys

Sixty percent of jockeys reported episodes of bingeing, usually after a race, in one study. Use of laxatives, diuretics and other dangerous weight control methods are common among male jockeys who are required to maintain a low weight for competition.

Bodybuilders

Bodybuilding and strength training for women is increasingly popular. Garner and Rosen suggest that its popularity may be "little more than a minor variation on the standard exploitive doctrine on the virtues of thinness and weight loss." Needed research is lacking in this area, they say.

However, it is unwarranted to conclude that athletes with disordered eating are suffering from the serious personality disturbances seen in most patients with anorexia nervosa or bulimia nervosa, even when weight-preoccupied, say the specialists. They may still be at risk, though, because heightened concerns about eating, weight and shape likely precede the development of severe eating disorders in most cases, and they may be at risk for developing eating disorders.

Runners

Among elite female runners, one study found 13 percent had reported a history of anorexia nervosa, and 34 percent indicated disturbed eating patterns consistent with those found in eating disorders. Another found that women who spent more hours per week jogging had more eating disorder symptoms. This does not answer the question of whether women with excessive concerns about weight choose these sports, or whether dedicating oneself to strenuous exercise may promote increased concerns about weight, shape and dieting, say Garner and Rosen.

An overlap exists between runners who are obsessed with weight loss to improve performance, and anorectics who exercise excessively in pursuit of thinness.

Gymnasts

A survey of 182 female college athletes in several sports found that potentially dangerous weight control behaviors were common. Fourteen percent reported that they used self-induced vomiting. Sixteen percent used laxatives to control weight. Among the gymnasts nearly 53 percent reported vomiting and 37 percent used laxatives. In another study of 42 female college gymnasts, cited by Garner and Rosen, all were trying to lose weight, and 25 percent had used vomiting for this purpose.

Sometimes coaches or trainers urge their athletes to lose weight – a dangerous practice, say eating disorder specialists. In one study of collegiate women gymnasts, 67 percent reported being told by their coaches they were too heavy and 75 percent of them had used hazardous methods to try to control their weight, including vomiting, laxative or diuretic abuse.

Olympic female gymnasts are being required to be younger, smaller and thinner year by year. The preferred weight by judges is now under 90 pounds, with body fat of less than 10 percent. Preferred age is 16 or

Olympic female gymnasts are younger, smaller and thinner. Preferred weight is under 90 pounds.

under, and height of girls who win has dropped to 4-feet-10 or under. The girls exchange stunted growth and a likely eating disorder for the privilege of competing as Olympic gymnasts, charges the American Anorexia/Bulimia Association.[3]

One who made the ultimate sacrifice for her sport was Christy Henrich, a world class gymnast who died in 1994 in Kansas City. Henrich said her dieting frenzy began in 1988 after a judge in an international Hungarian competition told her she needed to watch her weight. At that time she weighed 93 pounds and was at the height of her career. Christy Henrich died at age 22, weighing only 60 pounds.

Wrestlers

Wrestling is a sport on which much weight-related research has focused because of serious concerns of parents, teachers and coaches about the "weight cutting" behavior of high school wrestlers.

"If there's a way to lose weight, a wrestler will find it," said Don Herrmann, associate director of the Wisconsin Interscholastic Athletic Association. "I've seen self-induced vomiting, laxative abuse, excessive water and food deprivation, even a self-induced bloody nose."

A typical example is Cory Crawford, a 1991 graduate of Watertown (Wis.) High School, who weighed 156 before the start of his senior wrestling season, lost 11 pounds to wrestle at 145, and then decided with his coach to drop down to the 135-pound class to have a better chance at the state championship.

"On the day of the meet, I'd be one or two pounds over, so I'd run and I'd spit into a cup," said Crawford. "After a meet I'd eat, then come in on Monday at 140, 142, which is good because I could lose two to three pounds a night in time to get down for a meet on Thursday. You could lose it from sweating in practice, or some kids would go into a bathroom (where it's hotter) and jump rope. There'd be nights I'd lose only a half pound, or on a good night I could lose six."

A Pennsylvania study of 368 high school wrestlers found that 42 percent had lost 11 to 20 pounds at least once in their lives. One-fourth were losing 6 to 10 pounds every week. After a match 30 to 40 percent reported being preoccupied with food and eating out of control. The wrestlers used a variety of aggressive methods to lose weight, including dehydration, food restriction, fasting, vomiting, laxatives and diuretics. "Making weight" was associated with fatigue, anger and anxiety.[4]

"When you see a youngster playing defensive halfback at 165 on Thanksgiving and then in three weeks he's wrestling at 145 pounds, there's something wrong," says Roy Schleicher, associate director of the New Jersey State Interscholastic Athletic Association.

How does a wrestler lose weight?

Weight loss methods of college wrestlers were investigated with 42 college wrestlers by Suzanne Nelson Steen, MS, RD, and Shortie McKinney, PhD, RD.[5]

Most were using the techniques of reducing and depriving food, dehydration, and strenuous exercise in daily training sessions.

Steen and McKinney analyzed food intake at midseason, and a month before and after season. This included a four-day period extending two days before the match until the day after.

> *"If there's a way to lose weight, a wrestler will find it. I've seen vomiting, laxative abuse, even a self-induced bloody nose."*
> — Don Herrmann

During the season 37 percent of wrestlers did not meet the recommended dietary allowance (RDA) for calories. This is more severe, it is pointed out, because RDA does not account for their strenuous training activity. At the level of two thirds of RDA: one-quarter did not meet the criteria for vitamin C, iron, and thiamine, half did not meet it for vitamin A, and more than half for vitamin B6, magnesium, and zinc. Diets tended to be higher in fat and lower in carbohydrate than recommended.

Intake was extremely variable. For example, a 118-pound wrestler ate 334 calories the day before the match, 4,214 calories in the evening after his match, and 5,235 the next day. His weekly loss and regain were each 12 pounds.

Food and fluid intake was typically minimal and sometimes zero for both days previous to the match.

In the allotted five hours between weigh-in and match, fluid and food were increased in an attempt to rehydrate and restore strength, but the researchers say this is insufficient time for restoring electrolyte balance or replenishing muscle glycogen concentration. They suggest many wrestlers compete with greatly reduced carbohydrate stores, leading to premature fatigue and poor performance.

Among the wrestlers' nutrition misconceptions was the common view that starchy carbohydrates are fattening. One third avoided breads, pasta and potatoes.

They reported cravings for sweets when dieting.

After the season, their fat intake was considerably higher than either preseason or midseason, suggesting that perhaps deprivation increased preference for fat. Nutrition was generally adequate before and after the season.

Athletic trainers say that rapid weight loss for wrestlers can cause kidney and heart strain, low blood volume, electrolyte imbalances, increased irritability, depression, an inability to concentrate, and an increased vulnerability to eating disorders.[6]

Dehydration

A high percent of the wrestlers used dehydration techniques. These included saunas (51 percent), wrestling in a heated room (74 percent), wearing rubber or plastic suits while exercising (42 percent), and restricting drinking (58 percent). On one team 5 percent of the wrestlers used laxatives and diuretics, and 11 percent used vomiting to lose weight, all hazardous practices.

It is ironic, say Steen and McKinney, that 83 percent of the wrestlers correctly believed their sudden weight loss affected their performance. They cite research showing that after a 4 percent loss of body weight from dehydration, muscle endurance drops 31 percent for isometric and 29 percent for isotonic exercise. Even four hours after rehydration, endurance was as much as 21 percent below initial levels.

Competing while dehydrated is seen as an extremely hazardous practice which not only impairs muscle performance, but can inhibit sweating and increase risk of temperature regulation problems and heat stroke.

A call for 7% body fat

Wisconsin is a leader in raising body fat requirements for wrestlers

Among college gymnasts nearly 53 percent reported vomiting and 37 percent used laxatives.

to 7 percent, and in working to solve weight loss abuse problems in high school wrestling programs.[7]

In 1991, following a trial of pilot programs, Wisconsin adopted a minimum wrestling weight of 7 percent body fat for males and 12 percent for females, based on skinfold measurements by trained certified measurers. The new rules permit a 3 percent allowance. Thus, if a wrestler's predicted weight is 115 pounds, he will be able to wrestle at 112 pounds, but would be encouraged to wrestle at 119 instead.

A wrestler is not allowed to wrestle in a weight class for which he would need to lose more than three pounds a week from the original date of his measurement. Growth allowance is reinstated, with two additional pounds allowed for each weight class on Dec. 25, and one more pound on Feb. 1. The program also includes a nutrition education program in which a nutritionist trained in an understanding of the sport meets with wrestlers, coaches and parents.

Herrmann reports there is overwhelming support and enthusiasm for the new program. "Probably 60 percent of wrestling coaches openly opposed it in the early stages – they said we didn't need it, skinfold measures aren't accurate enough, and it would bring too much attention to wrestling weight concerns. There's been a dramatic swing in acceptance. Now 97 to 98 percent are in favor of it." He says coaches of other sports in the state want to be included in similar programs.

Recommendations in all states should be changed to raise body fat requirements from 5 to 7 percent for wrestlers, says Charles Tipton, PhD, in the *Physician and Sportsmedicine*. He cites a study of elite high school wrestlers at the Iowa State Wrestling Championships which found 30 percent of athletes tested had 5 percent or less body fat.[8]

The average young man carries about 14 to 16 percent body fat, but will likely strive for 5 to 7 percent if he is serious about sports in which leanness can be a factor, according to the U.S. Olympic Committee's Division of Sport Medicine and Science. Most young women have body fat of 20 to 22 percent, and many serious young female athletes strive for 5 to 7 percent body fat. Most authorities maintain that 5 percent body fat is the minimum at which an athlete can compete and still be healthy.

There is overwhelming evidence, Tipton says, that calorie restriction will ultimately diminish muscle strength and markedly reduce endurance. While student athletes need at least 1,500 to 2,200 calories per day, he says, they often eat between zero and 500 calories on days before a match.

Discussing the medical aspects of wrestling, four specialists in wrestling research cited in the report, express a strong concern for the abuses seen in the sport of wrestling. One warns that a sign of a wrestler losing too much weight is his loss of concentration – "a skinny kid walking around in a daze."

Another cites a study that found 7 percent of wrestlers use vomiting on a monthly basis, and 1 to 3 percent used diuretics or laxatives.

The loss of three or four pounds is big loss for the smaller wrestler, compared with the same amount for a 180-pounder, but it is often treated as the same by the coach.

The error factor of 5 to 7 percent, in even the best methods of testing body fat, is seen as a real problem, especially for the 103-pound wrestler.

Wisconsin requires a minimum wrestling weight of 7 percent body fat for males and 12 percent for females.

More accurate testing of body fat, and dehydration through urine tests is suggested. More extensive use of certified athletic trainers and nutritionists, to minimize the negative effects of weight-cutting, is also needed.[8]

Amenorrhea

Menstrual dysfunction and amenorrhea are common among female athletes in a wide range of sports, and severe weight restrictions may be one reason why. Suboptimal weight required for ballet has been linked to menstrual disturbance including delayed menarche and amenorrhea. These disturbances are associated with scoliosis and stress fractures in young ballet dancers.

Delayed puberty is also associated with higher activity levels and thinness for girls age 10 to 14. The age of menarche in the U.S. has dropped from age 15 or 16 in the past 100 years to an average age of 12.8, along with a childhood decrease in activity and increase in body fat. This drop is associated with high teenage pregnancy rates and higher reproductive cancer risk.

On the other hand, delayed menarche, which can be as late as age 19 or 20 for very thin female athletes and ballet dancers, is linked to osteoporosis and bone fractures.[9]

Eating disorder prevention

It is recommended that when even mild signs of eating disorders are observed in athletes, they should be given immediate attention. It is a mistake to assume the problem will correct itself, or to think that addressing the issues directly might reinforce the disordered behavior, say Garner and Rosen.

"The affected athlete often is struggling with the dilemma of wanting help and at the same time not wanting to reveal anything that may jeopardize his or her standing on the team," they explain.

Confounding the need for help may be the athlete's denial and secrecy.

If an eating disorder is suspected, it is recommended the coach or trainer with the best rapport with that athlete arrange a private meeting with her or him, giving support and offering help, while assuring confidentiality. The adult should approach the athlete directly, and not discuss suspected problems with teammates, say specialists.

It is vital for the athlete to understand that assistance is available and can help her or him to achieve or maintain success in the sport. In referrals, it is important for the clinician to have a good understanding of the demands of the sport as well as of eating disorders.

In some cases it is suggested that coaches and trainers may themselves have eating difficulties and destructive weight attitudes which are being conveyed to athletes. In this case, others may need to confront them to address these issues.

Puberty has dropped for girls from age 15 or 16 to 12.8 in the past 100 years. This drop is linked to high teenage pregnancy rates and cancer risk.

7. Eating disorders – physical and mental effects

"What is normal and what is disordered, for girls growing up in a culture that forces them to live as if their bodies are being constantly watched, desired and judged."

Some specialists are suggesting that dieting itself is a cause of the increase in eating disorders in the United States today, and that what is being called *chronic dieting syndrome* (frequent weight loss attempts followed by bingeing) should be treated and prevented. The current high rates of eating disorders are believed by many to be the inevitable result of 60 to 80 million Americans dieting, losing weight, rebounding, and learning to be chronic dieters.[1]

"Eating disorders should be called 'dieting disorders,' because it is the dieting process and not eating that causes the initiation of both anorexia nervosa and bulimia nervosa," says Joe McVoy, an eating disorder specialist at Springwood Hospital in Leesburg, Va.

McVoy says the term 'eating disorders' seems to indicate something is wrong with the eating process, whereas what happens is a conscious choice to restrict one's food intake or diet, which leads to starvation and ultimately the disorder.

Most professionals agree that dieting precedes the onset of an eating disorder. In fact, dieting is suggested as an important step in the progression from weight dissatisfaction to binge eating. A binge may be the natural and nearly inevitable result of food deprivation.

Many of the physical and mental abnormalities of eating disorders are common to chronic dieters and to people on severely restrictive diets. Many of the effects are typical of those described in Third World starvation conditions. Restoring full nutrition can bring dramatic improvement to both the mind and body.

While only a minority of people who diet develop eating disorders, some dieters may be more vulnerable than others. Factors that increase a dieter's vulnerability to eating disorders can be genetic, biological, psychological, personality, sociocultural and familial. Violence, trauma and childhood sexual abuse are considered to be risk factors. The National Women's Study finds women with bulimia nervosa about twice as likely to have been raped (26.6 vs 13.3 percent) or sexually molested (22 vs 12 percent), and four times as likely to have experienced aggravated assault (26.8 vs 8.4 percent) as women who have other psychiatric disorders but not an eating disorder. The majority report some type of criminal victimization event, compared with less than one-third (54.4 vs 31 percent) of the women without an eating disorder.[2] (Abuse is a risk factor for psychiatric disturbance.)

The traditional, patriarchal view suggests the roots for eating disorders lie with psychological traits of patients and their families.

Yet in less than two decades, the acceptable female body size has been whittled down by one-third, say Patricia Fallon, Melanie Katzman and Susan Wooley, editors of *Feminist Perspectives on Eating Disorders*.[3] Most women no longer fit that size, and trying to do so takes up more and more of their lives. Some are pushed to an apparent point of no return, say these eating disorder authorities, by "our era's culminating demand that women give up nourishment and a large share of their bodies."

Is something wrong in our culture that promotes what some have called an "epidemic" in eating disorders? That allows high rates of violence and sexual assault on women, at the same time it makes impossible demands for the attractiveness of the female body?

There appears to be a continuum of disordered eating among modern women, in the broader view expressed by eating disorder specialists Fallon, Katzman and Wooley. Women with fully developed eating disorders may be expressing what many other women are feeling.

What is "normal" and what is "disordered," for girls growing up in a culture that forces them to live as if their bodies are being constantly "watched, desired and judged," and that encourages them to use "the power of weakness."

An "epidemic" illness?

According to the National Eating Disorders Organization, anorexia nervosa affects about 1 in 500 adolescents (0.2 percent), 90 to 95 percent of them female.[4] Some studies find as many as 1 in 100 girls between 12 and 18 years (1 percent) are affected. Follow-up studies show death rates as high as 18 percent for anorexia nervosa and bulimia nervosa, report Dan Reiff and Kathleen Kim Lampson Reiff.[5]

Bulimia nervosa affects 1 to 3 percent of adolescents, according to the *Diagnostic and Statistical Manual*, 1994, American Psychiatric Association. A recent study of college freshmen found 4.5 percent of females and 0.4 percent of males had a history of bulimia nervosa, say the Reiffs.

Eating disorders are estimated to affect up to 7 percent of community populations and 10 percent of student populations. Approximately 9,000 patients are hospitalized annually in the U.S. for the treatment of eating disorders, according to Robin Sesan.[6]

Eating disorders are often associated with alcohol and/or drug abuse, which can increase the medical and mental complications.

One of the fastest growing eating disorder behaviors in the past five years is excessive exercise or exercise addiction to lose weight or sculpt the body, says McVoy. This entails exercise with the sole end of reducing calories or getting rid of body fat to change body appearance. Body sculpting basically means reducing body fat to as little as possible, so that the muscles can be more clearly defined, he says.

"This has become more epidemic because of the growth in our society of an emphasis on fitness and body shaping. There's a great increase in fitness magazines, fitness spas, and home exercise equipment all with a focus on shape and muscle building.

McVoy says the great increase in eating disorders in males appears to be growing out of this obsession with fitness and body sculpting. It reflects a dissatisfaction with one's natural body and an intense desire to change it.

Anorexia nervosa

Common signs and symptoms of eating disorders are fatigue, lethargy, weakness, impaired concentration, nonfocal abdominal pain, dizziness, faintness, sore muscles, chills, "cold sweat," frequent sore throats, diarrhea and constipation, according to Allan Kaplan and Paul Garfinkel

The great increase in eating disorders in males appears to be growing out of an obsession with fitness and body sculpting.

Thin people are the 'saints' among us
by Margaret Visser

The prestige that accrues to being thin arises from the difficulty of the enterprise, but also from its perversity. As an image and a metaphor, a strikingly thin body expresses, yet simultaneously flies in the face of, much that our culture idealizes. It suggests mobility, youth, self-control, and general toughness.

But it also symbolically contradicts the consumerism, the dedication to riches and growth, the proud capacity for incorporating everything from material resources to people and ideas . . .

Thin people, in other words, are walking paradoxes – having, yet metaphorically disowning, what everybody wants and envies.

The thin among us are the saints of the system; they fulfill our ideals while demonstrating impressive dedication and willpower in the process; their physical shape constitutes proof of guiltlessness.[51]

Reprinted from the Journal of Gastronomy.

in *Medical issues and the Eating Disorders.*[7]

In anorexia nervosa, the individual is more than 15 percent under expected weight, fears gaining weight, is preoccupied with food, has amenorrhea (or if male, a decrease in sexual drive or interest) and abnormal eating habits. There are two types: one simply restricts food, the other either purges alone or binges and purges regularly. Changes occur in behavior, perception, thinking, mood and social interaction. A sense of heightened control and control over food seems important to the person with anorexia nervosa. Pleasure and enjoyment during eating are replaced by guilt, anxiety and ambivalence. Mood tends to be depressed, irritable, anxious and unstable often leading to increased social isolation.

For anorexia nervosa the symptoms are usually obvious: emaciated appearance, dry skin, sometimes yellowish, fine body hair, brittle hair and nails, body temperature below 96.6 F, pulse rate usually below 60 beats per minute, subnormal blood pressure, and sometimes edema, say Kaplan and Garfinkel. Initially, these are symptoms associated with severely restrictive dieting: irritability, lightheadedness, hunger and decrease in energy, say the Reiffs. Then the consequences of prolonged semi-starvation begin to set in. Duration of the disorder may range from a single episode to a lifelong illness.

Bulimia nervosa

The person with bulimia nervosa goes on an eating binge at least twice a week, eating a very large amount of food within a discrete period, and then tries to compensate for this either by purging or nonpurging behavior. Some binge and purge many times a day. As the disorder progresses it develops into a complex lifestyle that is increasingly isolating from social relationships, with feelings of isolation, depressed mood and low self-esteem. In bulimic patients, vomiting is the most common form of purging. Up to one-third of anorexic individuals develop bulimia nervosa.

Patients with bulimia may seem physically healthy, but evidence of vomiting behavior may be present: finger calluses or lesions on the dominant hand from stimulating the gag reflex (especially in early stages when stimulation is needed to induce vomiting), puffy or "chipmunk" cheeks from stimulation of the salivary glands, erosion of enamel especially on the surface of the upper teeth next to the tongue.[8] The consequences of the self-abusive purging behavior become increasingly obvious as the frequency and duration increase, and include hair loss, fatigue, insomnia, muscle weakness, edema, dizziness, sore throat, stomach pain or cramping, bloating, bad breath and bloodshot eyes.

Other eating disorders

Another more general category is called *Eating disorders not otherwise specified,* and includes the newly listed *Binge Eating Disorder.* In this category are individuals who have severe eating disorders which for one reason or another do not fit the other two diagnostic criteria. They may be similar to anorexic or bulimic patients but lack one of the diagnostic criteria to fit those categories. Or they may repeatedly chew and spit out, but do not swallow, large amounts of food. The binge eating disorder meets the criteria for bulimia nervosa but individuals do not regularly engage in purging behaviors and are not unduly concerned with weight and shape. They may be average weight, but most often are obese.

Anorexia nervosa

Patients with anorexia nervosa refuse to maintain weight at or above what is minimally normal for age and height (less than 85% of expected weight), and have an intense fear of weight gain or becoming fat. They have disturbance in body image, causing undue influence on self-esteem. If female, they have amenorrhea, defined as the absence of at least three consecutive menstrual cycles.

Two types are:

● **Restricting type:** severely restrict food without regularly binge eating or purging.
● **Binge eating/purging type:** with binge eating or purging (induced vomiting or misuse of laxatives, diuretics or enemas).

See: Diagnostic criteria for eating disorders. Diagnostic and Statistical Manual, Fourth Edition, 1994. American Psychiatric Association, Washington, DC.

Medical complications

Anorexia Nervosa

- **Electrolytes.** May be low in potassium, sodium, chloride, calcium, magnesium, and high or low bicarbonate. Electrolyte imbalance more likely when there is dehydration and/or purging.
- **Gastrointestinal.** Constipation is likely, may promote laxative use. Commonly there is vomiting, feelings of fullness and bloating, and abdominal discomfort. There may be ulcers, and pancreatic dysfunction. Excessive laxatives over time may result in gastrointestinal bleeding and impairment of colonic functioning.
- **Cardiovascular.** Commonly present are chest pain, arrhythmias, hypotension, edema and mitral valve prolapse. Electrocardiogram (EKG) changes. Heart rates lower than 40 beats per minute are common and as low as 25 reported in severe starvation. Prolonged QT intervals can lead to sudden death syndrome.
- **Metabolic.** Abnormal temperature regulation and cold intolerance are common. Abnormal glucose tolerance, fasting hypoglycemia, high B-hydroxybutyric acid, high free fatty acids, hypercholesterolemia, hypercarotenemia are common. Diabetic patients with an eating disorder may have fluctuating blood glucose levels leading to serious longterm consequences.
- **Bones.** Decreased bone mineral density may lead to fractures, growth retardation, short stature and osteoporosis.
- **Renal.** Elevated blood urea nitrogen, changes in urinary concentration capacity, and decreased glomerular filtration rate are common.
- **Endocrine.** Amenorrhea is 100%, by definition, although many anorexia nervosa patients begin to menstruate over time. Related to weight loss but may precede weight loss (in one-third); may cause delayed puberty, contributes to osteoporosis, breast atrophy, infertility. Hypometabolic state resulting in cold intolerance, dry skin and hair, bradycardia, constipation, fatigue, slowed reflexes. High plasma cortisol, decreased cortixol response to insulin.
- **Hematologic.** Anemia, leukopenia, bone marrow hypocellularity, common; these effects are usually mild, but can include bleeding tendency.
- **Neurological.** EEG and sleep changes are common; epileptic seizures affect up to 10 percent.
- **Musculocutaneous.** Muscle weakening, muscle cramps. Hair loss, brittle hair and nails, lanugo hair, dry skin and cold extremities are common.

(Source: Medical issues and the Eating Disorders)[9]

Bulimia nervosa

- **Electrolytes.** Low potassium, low chloride, dehydration and metabolic alkalosis are common. May lead to cardiac arrest, renal failure. Dehydration is common along with hypotension, dizziness, weakness, muscle cramps. Cardiac arrhythmias affect 20 percent; unpredictable, may require emergency treatment. Hypochloremia is common; limits kidney's ability to excrete bicarbonate.
- **Gastrointestinal.** Constipation and increased amylase common. Rarely gastric and duodenal ulcer, acute gastric dilation and rupture.

Bulimia nervosa

In bulimia nervosa the individual has recurrent episodes of binge eating. An episode includes eating, in a discrete period of time, an amount of food larger than most people would eat, and a sense of lack of control over what or how much one is eating during the episode. It includes recurrent inappropriate compensatory behavior to prevent weight gain, such as induced vomiting, misuse of laxatives, diuretics, enemas, or other medications; fasting; or excessive exercise. Both binge eating and the compensatory behavior occur at least twice a week for three months, on average. One's self-evaluation is unduly influenced by body shape and weight. (The disturbance does not occur exclusively during episodes of anorexia nervosa.)

Two types are:
- **Purging type:** uses regular purging behavior (induced vomiting or misuse of laxatives, diuretics or enemas).
- **Nonpurging type:** uses other inappropriate compensatory behaviors, such as fasting or excessive exercise, but does not regularly engage in purging.

See: Diagnostic criteria for eating disorders. Diagnostic and Statistical Manual, Fourth Edition, 1994. American Psychiatric Association, Washington, DC.

Frequent abdominal pain. Severe abdominal pain may lead to rigid abdomen and shock which may result in death. Abuses of laxatives may lead to iron deficiency anemia, rectal bleeding and cathartic colon.

- **Pulmonary.** Aspiration pneumonia possible from aspiration of vomitus.

- **Cardiovascular.** Peripheral edema is common along with EKG changes and QT changes, which can lead to serious arrhythmias and congestive heart failure. Uncommon is sudden cardiac death. Ipecac syrup abuse may lead to death through cardiomyopathy, myocarditis.

- **Metabolic.** High B-hydroxybutyric acid, free fatty acids. Less common edema, abnormal temperature regulation and cold intolerance.

- **Renal.** Possible changes.

- **Endocrine.** Menstrual irregularities with low body weight, dexamethasone nonsuppression common.

- **Hematologic.** May be anemic with nutrition deficiency.

- **Neurological.** EEG changes common. May have epileptic seizures with malnutrition and electrolyte imbalance.

- **Musculocutaneous.** Calluses on dorsum of dominant hand are common from inducing gag reflex. Muscle weakening with ipecac abuse.

- **Dental.** Enamel erosions with vomiting.

(Source: Medical issues and the Eating Disorders)

Psychological profiles
Anorexia Nervosa

Many of the mental and emotional symptoms common to anorexia nervosa are directly related to the physical effects of starvation. These are documented in the wartime Keys Minnesota Starvation Study in which 32 men underwent dramatic personality changes during six months on half rations, when they lost one-fourth of their weight. Other traits have to do with attitudes and behavior toward eating and weight. The following are psychological traits commonly associated with anorexia nervosa.[10]

- **Energy level.** Fatigue, weakness, lassitude, lethargy, apathy, decreasing energy, persistent tiredness dizziness, faintness, lightheadedness, yet compulsively exercises (hyperactive).

- **Mood, attitude and behavior.** Moodiness, often depressed or irritable, mood swings (tyrannical); anxiety and ambivalence; irritability; critical; less tolerant of others; depression; low self-esteem, self-esteem control through weight loss; invulnerability and success dependent on weight loss; feelings of lack of control in life; hopelessness; rigidity, highly controlled behavior; does not reveal feelings; perfectionist behavior; fantasy that weight loss can cause or prevent some life event (prevent parental divorce, attract romance); denies hunger; denies problem of weight loss (sees self as fat); denies eating disorder; body image distortion (overestimates body size and shape, "feels fat" despite emaciated appearance);

Eating disorder not otherwise specified

The third and largest eating disorder category is *Eating disorder not other wise specified*. Individuals in this category do not meet the definitions for either anorexia nervosa or bulimia nervosa.

Examples are:

- All criteria met for anorexia nervosa except amenorrhea.
- All criteria met for anorexia nervosa except, despite weight loss, current weight is in normal range.
- All criteria met for bulimia nervosa except frequency of binges is less than twice a week or for a duration of less than three months.
- An individual of normal body weight who regularly engages in inappropriate compensatory behavior (such as induced vomiting) after eating small amounts of food
- Repeatedly chewing and spitting out large amounts of food, without swallowing.
- Binge eating disorder.

See: Diagnostic criteria for eating disorders. Diagnostic and Statistical Manual, Fourth Edition, 1994. American Psychiatric Association, Washington, DC.

ritualistic habits.

- **Mental ability.** Inability to concentrate, decreased alertness; difficulty with reading comprehension, diminished capacity to think; loss of memory; extreme narrowing of interests; decline in ambition.

- **Social.** Social withdrawal, isolates self from family and friends, becomes increasingly aloof and withdrawn; loneliness; feelings easily hurt; avoidance by peers; worsening family relations, fights with family, cost of treatment may be financial drain.

- **Weight.** increasing preoccupation with body; frequently monitors body changes (may check with scale and/or mirror many times per day); compares size and shape to others, envious of thinner persons; heightened control, feelings of having control over body.

- **Food, eating and hunger.** Misperception of hunger, satiety and other bodily sensations; hunger and increasing hunger; fears food and gaining weight; eats alone; guilt when eating; may secretly binge; dieting and weight increasingly important focus; unusual food-related behaviors (makes rules for specific foods, placement on plate, time of eating, size of bites, number of chews per bite); progressive preoccupation with food and eating (may begin to cook and control family's eating); need to vicariously enjoy food (may collect recipes, dream of food, hoard food, enjoy watching others eat, pursue food-related careers – as dietitians, chefs, caterers).

- **Other.** Hypersensitive to cold and heat, hypersensitive to noise and light; sleep disturbance.

Bulimia nervosa

When a patient with anorexia becomes bulimic, she experiences symptoms characteristic of both eating disorders. The woman with bulimia nervosa is often of normal weight and may not experience the effects of starvation. However, if she has severe nutrition deficiencies due to purging, she may have some of the same starvation symptoms.

Typically, these mental and emotional symptoms may be associated with bulimia nervosa:

- **Mood/attitude/behavior.** Anxiety, depression; mood swings; low self-esteem, self-deprecating thoughts; embarrassment, shame related to behavior; persistent remorse; paranoid feelings; unreasonable resentments; makes excuses to go to restroom after meals; may buy large amounts of food, which suddenly disappears, impulsive as compared to anorexics who are overcontrolled.

- **Mental ability.** Loss of ordinary willpower, poor impulse control, self-indulgent behavior; recognizes abnormal eating behavior.

- **Social.** Depends on others for approval; feelings of isolation; unable to discuss problem, others unhappy about food obsession; social isolation; distancing friends and family; fear of going out in public; family, work and money problems.

- **Weight.** Feels that self worth is dependent on low weight; constant concern with weight and body image.

- **Food, eating and hunger.** Eats alone; eats when not hungry; preoc-

---

Binge eating disorder

Binge eating disorder is a subtype under the category *Eating disorder not otherwise specified.* It is defined as recurrent episodes of binge eating, which includes eating, in a discrete period of time, an amount of food larger than most people would eat, and a sense of lack of control over eating it. The individual has marked distress regarding binge eating, and engages in binge eating on average, at least 2 days a week for 6 months. (The binge eating is not associated with the regular use of inappropriate compensatory behaviors and does not occur exclusively during the course of anorexia nervosa or bulimia nervosa.)

At least three of the following must be part of the binge episode:

- Eating much more rapidly than normal.
- Eating until uncomfortably full.
- Eating large amounts of food when not hungry.
- Eating alone because of embarrassment about how much is eaten.
- Feeling disgusted with oneself, depressed, or very guilty about eating.

See: Diagnostic criteria for eating disorders. Diagnostic and Statistical Manual, Fourth Edition, 1994. American Psychiatric Association, Washington, DC.

It may be healthier to suggest acceptance; prevent future weight gain, stop binge eating.

— ADA

cupation with eating and food; fears binges and eating out of control; increased dependency on bingeing; binge eating of large amount of food in a short time, feeling out of control, cannot stop eating.

• **Purging.** Feels need to rid body of calories consumed during binge (through vomiting, laxatives, diuretics, enemas, fasting or excessive exercise); experimentation with vomiting, laxatives and diuretics often leads to regular abuse.

• **Binge/purge cycle.** Spends much time planning, carrying out, cleaning up after bulimic episode; eliminates normal activities; complex lifestyle may develop with episodes occurring several times a day; worsening of symptoms during times of emotional stress; feels soothed and comforted by binge/purge cycle – it may serve to relieve frustration, anxiety, anger, fear, remorse, boredom, loneliness.

• **Other.** Dishonesty, lying; stealing food or money; drug and alcohol abuse; suicidal tendencies or attempts.

ADA warns against weight loss promotion

Many persons with Binge Eating Disorder or other eating disorders seek weight loss treatment; however, this can be very detrimental to their physical and mental health, the American Dietetic Association warns in a 1994 position paper on treating eating disorders.

The position paper tells dietitians that many women may benefit more from counseling about body image issues and how to stop the pursuit of thinness than from weight loss itself.

Therefore, instead of providing weight loss treatment, it may be healthier to suggest accepting themselves at or near their present weight, learning how to prevent future weight gain, and stopping binge eating. Educating the lay public and other health professionals to help prevent eating disorders is important, says the ADA position paper.

8. Psychological risks

The psychological damage that can be inflicted by this national emphasis on weight loss and dieting is drawing closer scrutiny today. Yet, social costs have scarcely been recognized.

Americans have a compelling fear of fat, especially women. In record numbers women are trying to lose weight, often through self-starvation methods. As a result, many suffer permanent injury from malnutrition, and others are psychologically scarred.

At any given moment, about 40 percent of women and 25 percent of men are trying to lose weight, according to national studies.

In what is truly a national crisis, as many as 80 percent of girls age 10 and 11 have disordered eating behavior and are restricting their eating. It has become "the norm" for young girls.

The psychological costs of this epic struggle are high.

Yet it is critical that this nation consider not only the costs of widespread self-starvation to individuals, but what it is doing to the fabric of American society. How do the isolating effects of starvation alter careers and worksite relationships? What is it doing to parenting, to marital relations, to community service?

Dieting distorts development

"Dieting is not just about eating," warns Janet Polivy, PhD, a professor of psychology and psychiatry at the University of Tronoto who has researched dieting and its effects for nearly 20 years. "It is an entire way of life. Life has a different meaning for people when they become dieters. Their self-image and self-esteem is all tied up in this."

Polivy says the dangers of dieting include emotional and psychological harm, eating disorders, financial cost, and diminished lifestyle.

Her research shows dieters respond differently than non-dieters in a range of situations. Chronic dieters are easily upset, emotional, have mood swings, are more likely to eat when anxious, have trouble concentrating on the task at hand with any kind of distraction, can go longer without food and eat less under "ideal" circumstances. But they binge or eat more once started, then experience guilt. They are compliant and have a need for perfection, are preoccupied with weight and body dissatisfaction, have lost touch with internal signals of hunger and satiety and rely on cognitive cues for eating. They salivate more when faced with attractive food, and have higher levels of digestive hormones and elevated levels of free fatty acids in their blood.

A chronic dieter focuses on food, eating and weight both for herself and in her perception of others, has low self-esteem, and is eager to please and do what others ask of her.

Polivy argues that dieting is causal to these factors.[1]

Never put a child on a diet, advises Ellyn Satter, RD, a childhood eating specialist in Wisconsin, and author of *How to Get Your Kid to Eat – But Not Too Much.* "Diets are not an option. Restricting food intake, even in indirect ways, profoundly distorts developmental needs of children and adolescents."

It's time to define problems of childhood obesity in ways they can be solved, rather than continuing to set patients up for failure, she says.

"Dieting is not just about eating. It is an entire way of life."

— Janet Polivy

Isolating effects

The isolating effects of severe dieting have much in common with the self-starvation of anorexia nervosa. Young women in the grip of anorexia nervosa turn inward, become self-absorbed and self-focused. They exhibit an array of neurotic personality traits which can disappear entirely when eating is fully restored. Psychological effects of eating disorders, detailed in Chapter 7 *(page 56-62)*, include apathy, moodiness, depression, inability to concentrate, narrowing of interests, social withdrawal, loneliness, anxiety and irritability.

Similarly, the Minnesota Experiment in human starvation, conducted in 1944 and 1945, documented profound personality changes, as well as physical changes, in the 32 men who for six months cut their daily energy intake to 1,570 calories, or about in half. Of the many changes, nearly all were detrimental to mental health.[2]

As starvation progressed, the men grew weak, nervous, anxious, apathetic and depressed. Their interests narrowed. They isolated themselves and increasingly spent time alone. As their heart size shrunk, metabolism slowed, and muscles weakened, many became neurotic and some behavior verged on being psychotic. The men became self-centered, sarcastic and argumentative, with little interest or concern for others. Personal appearance deteriorated. Sexual interest and fuction decreased.

This was a major change from their behavior during the initial control period. An idealistic, well-educated group, the men had been responsive, tolerant and good-humored. Many volunteered to help with overseas relief operations after the war. They developed a lively group spirit and laid plans for educational activities - plans which quietly fell apart under the stress of starvation.

More recently, anthropologist Colin Turnbull studied a starving society in the mountains of east Africa (Uganda, Kenya and the Sudan).[3] His book *The Mountain People* is a painful narrative about a band of Ik hunting people who were driven from their natural hunting grounds into a barren wasteland by the creation of a game refuge. They are forbidden to kill wild animals and ordered to farm in a land without rain. The social effects of starvation among these people are frightening.

According to his account, as starvation advanced each person turned inward, living in isolation, concerned only with obtaining food. Men and women went off alone to forage for food, finding it sometimes in scarce vegetation, or by following the flight of vultures to an animal carcass, or by watching others to discover hidden food caches. They returned empty-handed to avoid the risk of being robbed or the need to share with crying children, a sick spouse, or aged parents.

Turnbull reported a breakdown of the family unit. Parents expected children by the age of three to fend for themselves. They did not even bring water to their thirsty children. The old were abandoned. Children stole food from the mouths of their grandparents.

The Ik people feared and mistrusted each other, giving no word of encouragement to family members who were struggling or ill. In their lives cruelty took the place of love, Turnbull said, but each person was so isolated that "I do not think they thought of their cruelty as affecting others."

They laughed only at another's misfortune, which they seemed to

The social effects of starvation were frightening . . . each person turned inward, living in isolation, concerned only with obtaining food.

enjoy, such as when someone tripped or fell. There was a chill dispassionate regard of the cruelest of incidents. They seldom spoke or interacted with others. A total loss of sexual interest, Turnbull suggests, deprived the Ik of a major drive toward sociability, and jeopardized the continuation of their society.

Starvation led to complete moral breakdown of the culture, including loss of religion, rituals and spirituality, and the lack of any sense of moral obligation. They were a loveless people.

Thus, it becomes painfully clear that basic human qualities such as family, love, human kindness, generosity, neighborliness, and religious belief may become luxuries that do not concern the starving person, as she or he turns increasingly inward to a preoccupation with self alone.

At first glance, these studies may seem to have little relevance to modern society. How do they apply to a wealthy nation in which many women keep themselves in a state of self-starvation, not from necessity or a sense of self-sacrifice, but from a sole concern for the appearance of their own bodies?

Many women in America routinely live at a level far below the 1,570-calorie diet which caused such drastic personality changes for men in the Minnesota Experiment. By some estimates as many as 18 to 82 percent of young women have maladaptive eating behavior which includes severe restriction of food and fasting.[4] An estimated 18 percent of female students may have clinically defined eating disorders.

Undernourished children have diminished capacity to learn and this contributes to illiteracy in America, say Carl Sagan and Ann Druyan, authors of *Shadows of Forgotten Ancestors.*[5] Instead of showing an enthusiasm, a zest for learning – as most healthy youngsters do – the undernourished child becomes bored, apathetic, unresponsive. Iron-deficiency anemia, which may affect as many as one-fourth of all low-income children in America, attacks the attention span and memory, they report. Without doubt, it affects enormous numbers of chronically dieting women.

Starvation, in the quest for thinness as decreed by a corporate power structure, keeps women weak, preoccupied, passive and submissive, charges Naomi Wolf, author of *The Beauty Myth.*[6] And the public is silent when young women die, she notes.

Decline in generosity

One might even conclude that the apparent decline in volunteerism and the spirit of generosity which so long typified this country may result, in part, from the obsession with thinness.

Americans today hold high standards for physical appearance, confer high status on people with thin bodies, but are perhaps less neighborly than in the past.

Author Neal Gabler, writing in the Los Angeles Times, decries the narcissism of modern culture. "We have turned from the community to ourselves, from the common good to our own good, becoming fixated with our personal development, our material well-being, our emotional satisfaction. Certainly the '80s testified to that."[7]

Both the Minnesota Experiment and the anthropological study of the Ik hunters report antisocial behavior and self-absorption as a result of starvation. With this country's alarming rate of eating disorders and national preoccupation with thinness, it's perhaps not unrealistic to attribute some of today's social problems to the isolating effects of malnu-

"Starvation in the quest for thinness keeps women weak, preoccupied, passive and submissive."
— Naomi Wolf

trition and progressive self-starvation.

Modern researchers say that for humanitarian reasons, the Minnesota Experiment could never be repeated. But the statistics on weight loss and eating disorders suggest it is being repeated, without adequate controls, on large numbers of Americans at potentially staggering social, mental and emotional costs.

Many American women and men are each year subjected to similar experiments in university treatment centers and nonprofit clinics supported by public funds. Diets of 800 calories or less, lasting four to six months are not at all unusual in this research. Many such studies are reported in scientific journals. Unfortunately the scientific basis is often weak. For all the suffering they exact, the studies usually only focus on reporting short-term positive results of commerical programs. There is little or no documentation or recognition of possible adverse effects. Yet, it is critically important to know the full story of what is happening to these patients.

Healthy Weight Journal has challenged researchers to provide this information, to measure and report detrimental as well as beneficial effects, including mental, emotional and social effects, using objective standards in a scientific manner as did the Minnesota Experiment. As of 1995, this hasn't happened.

Below are the psychological effects found in the Minnesota Experiment in human starvation, as reported by Ancel Keys and colleages in *The Biology of Human Starvation:*

Personality changes

- Apathy, depression and tiredness increased.
- Irritability and moodiness increased.
- Self-discipline, mental alertness, comprehension and concentration decreased.
- Deterioration of spontaneous activity, including intellectual pursuits.
- Loss of ambition, a narrowing of interests.
- Feeling ineffective in daily living.
- The men felt distracted when they attempted to continue their cultural interests and studies. They were frustrated by the discrepancy between what they wanted to do and did do.
- They believed their judgment was impaired; however, tests showed this was unchanged, and they appeared to think clearly. (The researchers suggest this erroneous belief stemmed from feelings of apathy and narrowed interests).
- Decrease in sexual interest and loss of libido.
- Personal appearance and grooming deteriorated; the men often neglected to shave, brush their teeth, or comb their hair; they continued bathing, however, as one source of pleasure in feeling warm and relieving aches, pain and fatigue.
- An average rise toward the neurotic end of profile.
- Six subjects reacted to semi-starvation stress with severe "character neurosis." Two cases bordering on psychosis included vio-

They ate their food to the last crumb and licked their plates.

lence and hysteria.

- A rise in hysteria scores.
- Sensitivity to noise.
- Sometimes highly nervous, restless and anxious.
- The men carried out their chores and duties poorly.

Food preoccupation

- Increase in food interest; there was a preoccupation with food talk and food thoughts, though some subjects became annoyed by this in others.
- The men spent much time collecting recipes, studying cookbooks and menus, and fixing food saved from mealtime.
- An increased anticipation heightened their craving for food at meals.
- The men did much planning about how they would handle the day's allottment of food.
- Food dislikes disappeared. Taste appeal of the monotonous meals increased as time went on.
- The men became possessive about their food.
- They demanded that food and beverages be hot.
- They toyed with their food to make it seem like more and of greater variety. Often, toward the end, they would dawdle over a meal for two hours.
- For some there appeared a conflict in whether to stall out eating or ravenously gulp their food.
- The men became angry when they saw others wasting food.
- They ate their food to the last crumb and licked their plates.
- They did not dream of food, however, as some other reports have suggested.
- Extensive gum chewing; one man increased his gum chewing to 40 packs a day.
- Increased drinking of coffee and tea.
- The men increased their smoking, and some nonsmokers began smoking.
- Nail-biting, not seen in the initial control period, became common.
- The men became somewhat acquisitive in purchasing useless articles they could hardly afford and afterwards did not want; others became extremely anxious about saving money for "a rainy day."

Social activities

- Deterioration was seen in the group's spirit. During initial 12-week control period a group feeling had developed which was lively, responsive, tolerant and happy, with outstanding qualities of humor

The Minnesota Experiment is being repeated, without adequate controls, on large numbers of Americans at potentially staggering social, mental and emotional costs.

and high spirits. This gradually disappeared, and the tone became sober, serious, and what humor remained tended to be sarcastic.

- The men became reluctant to make group decisions or to plan activities, even though earlier they had taken an active interest in making policies and rules.

- They were reluctant to participate in group activities, saying it was too much trouble to contend with other people; they spent more time alone, became self-centered and egocentric.

- Social interaction seemed stilted, and politeness artificial.

- Food was the central topic of conversation; the men talked of little but hunger, food, weight loss, and their "guinea pig" way of life.

- The men were aware of their hyper-irritability, but were not entirely able to control emotionally charged responses, outbursts of temper, periods of sulking, and violence. Some men became scapegoats and targets of aggression for rest.

- Occasionally, exhilaration and feelings of well-being were brought on by such things as a variation in daily routine, lasting from a few hours to several days, but these were inevitably followed by "low" periods.

- Educational programs, which the men had organized to prepare themselves for anticipated careers in foreign relief work, quietly collapsed.

Refeeding

During the first six weeks of the refeeding period the men were divided into four groups, consuming 1,877 to 4,158 calories. At 13 weeks they were allowed free access to food. Refeeding effects were as follows:

- The men's spirits continued low for six weeks, and many were more depressed and irritable than ever.

- There was a slump in morale, and the men lost all interest in their earlier humanitarian concerns for the welfare of starving people.

- They became argumentative, and questioned the value of the experiment, as well as the competence of the researchers; they expressed feelings of being "let down." (This aggressiveness was seen by the researchers as evidence of increasing energy, and that the men were becoming less introverted and more interested in their environment.)

- Hunger pangs were reported as more intense than ever.

- During the first 12 weeks of rehabilitation, appetites were insatiable; all the men, including those on the highest calorie diets, wanted more food even when they were physically full.

- Many found it hard to stop eating, although "stuffed to bursting."

- The men were still concerned with food and their rations, above all else.

- They continued licking their plates, playing with food, and avoiding waste. Although this was a highly educated group, the men's table manners and eating habits had deteriorated, and during refeeding several deteriorated even more.

"We have turned from the community to ourselves, from the common good to our own good, becoming fixated with our personal development, our material well-being, our emotional satisfaction."

— Neal Gabler

- The urgent desire for dietary freedom was so extreme that postponing it another week produced severe emotional crisis and nearly open rebellion. All were counting the hours until they would have more food, even those who been eating 4,014 calories a day for two weeks.
- During week 13, when restrictions were lifted, the men ate an average of 5,218 calories per day. Their time was largely devoted to eating and sleeping, and they ate nearly continuously, eating as many as three consecutive lunches.
- By week 15, there was more social behavior at meals.
- By week 15, the table manners of 19 of 26 men were normal or nearly normal, but the other 7 still gobbled their food, had the desire to lick their plates and licked their knives when they could.
- Of 17 who left the laboratory, 15 reported they ate from 50 to 200 percent more than before the experiment and snacked often; one said he ate immense meals and then started snacking an hour after finishing a meal.
- By week 20, all said they felt nearly normal and were less preoccupied with food.
- By week 33, 10 of 14 who remained at the laboratory were eating normal amounts. The others ate more than before. One man, who ate 25 percent more and was gaining excess weight, tried to eat less but became so hungry he said he couldn't stand it and returned to excessive eating.
- Slowly humor, enthusiasm and sociability returned, and the men began looking forward to their plans for the future.

The tone became sober, serious, and what humor remained tended to be sarcastic.

9. Weight cycling

Heart disease and premature death were 25 to 100 percent more likely with high weight variability.

The possible risks of repeated bouts of losing and regaining weight, called weight cycling or yo-yo dieting, have gained wide attention in the public press. And for good reason: if weight cycling is harmful and is the almost inevitable result of weight loss, then perhaps weight loss itself is harmful and weight loss an inappropriate goal even for large patients, placing more importance on prevention.

This possibility has major implications for the $30 to $50 billion weight loss industry and for the focus of health care in the United States.

Weight cycling has been under intense investigation at several institutions in the U.S. and other countries since 1986, following studies that suggested losing weight on a very low calorie diet and regaining that weight made subsequent weight loss more difficult.[1]

However, research has shown inconsistent results on several issues. This has led some researchers to conclude weight cycling is not important. Others believe the variables have not yet been found which affect weight cycling changes – perhaps certain subgroups are more likely to be affected, or individuals are more vulnerable at times in their lives, such as during pregnancy.

The Diet and Health report of the National Academy of Sciences notes the possible detrimental effects of weight cycling. Similarly, the Surgeon General's Report on Nutrition and Health recommends that "the health consequences of repeated cycles of weight loss and gain" be given "special priority," and a poll of obesity experts lists weight cycling as one of the key causes of obesity.[2]

There is little doubt that weight cycling is extremely prevalent in the U.S. Sixty to 80 million people are trying to lose weight, and most of those who lose weight apparently regain it fairly quickly.

In a review of weight cycling research, Kelly Brownell and Judith Rodin cite a six-year study which tracked the weight of 153 middle-aged adults and found the women lost an average of 27 pounds and gained 31 pounds during the six years. The men lost and gained an average of more than 22 pounds. For the women, this was a gain of 21 percent of their initial body weight, and a loss of 19 percent. For the men it was about 12 percent lost and gained.

Another study tracked 332 overweight persons and found the vast majority either lost or gained significant amounts of weight.[3]

Weight cycling research focuses on two major issues:

1. Is weight cycling associated with increased risk to physical or mental health?
2. Does weight cycling make weight management more difficult by invoking survival mechanisms?

Major concerns have been raised that cycles of weight variability increase risk factors and the risk of mortality, especially cardiovascular deaths. Other concerns are that weight cycling may lower metabolic rate, decrease the ability to lose weight, increase the body's fat-to-lean ratio and waist-hip ratio, and increase the appetite for dietary fat.

Cycling may threaten heart

Research consistently shows an increase in mortality from all causes and from coronary heart disease with weight cycling.

Heart disease in men

Men who gain and lose large amounts of weight in middle adulthood may have a 26 percent increased risk for death from coronary heart disease after age 40, concluded researchers who re-analyzed data from the 1957 Western Electric Study.

Using the 1,957 subjects' self-reported weights from ages 20 to 40, they calculated the percentage change in weight every five years. The men fell into four groups: those who gained or lost 10 percent of their body mass index from one 5-year period to the next, those who gained 10 percent BMI in a 5-year period only, those who did not change weight, and the remainder.

Even after adjusting for age, serum cholesterol, blood pressure, cigarette smoking, alcohol consumption and body mass index, the risk for those in the gain and loss group remained twice as high as for those who experienced no change.[S1]

Weight cycling is associated with greater risks for coronary heart disease and other severe health problems in a major study published recently in the *New England Journal of Medicine* by L. Lissner and colleagues *(Figure1, page 74).*[4]

The findings are based on a 32-year analysis of weight fluctuations in 3,130 men and women in the Framingham Heart Study.

Individuals with a high weight variability – many weight changes or large changes – were 25 to 100 percent more likely to be victims of heart disease and premature death than those whose weight remained stable. They had increased total mortality, and increased mortality and morbidity due to coronary heart disease.

The relative risk for a high degree of weight variability compared with 1.0 for a low degree of variability is as follows:

Men
   Total mortality 1.30
   Mortality due to CHD..................1.48
   Morbidity due to CHD................1.48
   Morbidity due to cancer 1.04

Women
   Total mortality 1.27
   Mortality due to CHD..................1.47
   Morbidity due to CHD................1.42
   Morbidity due to cancer 1.16

These results seemed to hold true regardless of the individual's initial weight, long-term weight trend and/or cardiovascular risk factors such as blood pressure, cholesterol level, glucose tolerance, smoking and physical activity.

Even though nearly 50 percent of women who diet are not overweight, the researchers note, the weight cycling risks are seen at all weight categories, whether thin or obese.

The degree of weight variability was evaluated in relation to total mortality, mortality from coronary heart disease, morbidity due to coronary heart disease and morbidity due to cancer. Risks were considerably increased for all except cancer, which did not differ significantly.

When age groups were considered separately, weight fluctuation was most strongly associated with adverse health outcomes in the youngest group (age 30 to 40). This is also the group seen as most likely to diet.

The researchers found that a person's weight at age 25 makes an important contribution to whether there will be great variability.

Both men and women gained weight at an average rate of .11 kg per square meter per year.

Researchers from Goteborg, Sweden, and Boston University are involved in the current study. They cite their research in Sweden which found large fluctuations in body weight, measured at three intervals, was associated with heart disease in men and total mortality in both men and women.

In an effort to control for weight changes that may have been caused by illness, diseases and deaths for the first four years were excluded. This study does not distinguish between several weight changes and a single large weight change.

Weight cycling women

A history of repeated weight gain and loss, as well as pregnancy, may cause a higher waist-to-hip circumference ratio in women. A study of 87 pre-menopausal women between age 21 and 40 were measured for waist-hip ratio (WHR) and body mass index (BMI), and asked about magnitude and frequency of weight loss and pregnancy history.

Two groups were defined, one of weight cyclers and the other non-weight cyclers. Although mean BMIs were not significantly different (21.5 and 22.6), the WHR was higher among weight cyclers (.59) and self-reported "yo-yo dieters" (.75) than non-weight cyclers (.10).

However, another study of 846 middle-aged men from the Baltimore Longitudinal Study of Aging found that although weight fluctuation increased body fat centralization, the waist-hip ratio did not increase significantly.[52]

Weight cycling drops metabolism for wrestlers

Weight cycling is practiced with single-minded dedication by many high school and college athletes in the sport of wrestling.

Not only must the elite wrestler be talented, fit and superbly trained, but usually he is also actively engaged in weight reduction, even in the lower weight classes of 103 and 112 pounds.

The weight-cycling wrestler commonly loses 10 or more pounds in a few days to make weigh-ins for a match or tournament. He regains this weight quickly, and repeats the cycle many times throughout the wrestling season. Severe water deprivation and dehydration are often a part of his fasting episodes.

Long term effects of such strenuous weight loss efforts on the young wrestler are unknown.

Cold intolerance, weakness, and inability to concentrate are frequently reported. Other reported effects include changes in electrolyte balance, testosterone levels, nutritional status, renal function, thermal regulation, body composition and strength.

Growth and development may be delayed during one of the most active growth periods of a young man's life. The possibility of developing long-lasting eating disorders has been suggested.

Food efficiency

Metabolic effects of this severe weight cycling may cause an increase in food efficiency, and make losing more difficult.

Recent research with high school wrestlers on loss-and-gain cycles gives evidence of a lowered metabolism, as reported in the *Journal of the American Medical Association.*

The wrestlers were attending summer camp at the University of Iowa. It was several months after their last competitive match, and their weight had returned to normal.

The group of 27 wrestlers who cycled their weight were found to have significantly lower resting metabolic rate per unit of lean body mass than those defined as noncyclers.

Weight cyclers were defined as those who:
1. Cut weight 10 or more times during wrestling season.
2. Lost 4.5 kg or more weekly.
3. Reported they cut weight often or always.

Noncyclers:
1. Cut weight less than 5 times during the season.
2. Lost no more than 1.4 kg weekly.
3. Reported they cut weight sometimes, rarely or never.

Noncyclers were matched for age, weight, height, surface area, lean body mass, and percent body fat.

The cyclers competed farther below their natural off-season weight than did the noncyclers.

Results showed a significant difference in resting metabolic rate between the cyclers and noncyclers. The difference in resting energy expenditure was 14 percent. Oxygen consumption differed significantly. No differences were shown in respiratory quotient, oral temperature, pulse or blood pressure.

Studies needed

The researchers suggest weight cycling was a likely cause of lower metabolic rates, although they grant it is possible that low metabolism came first and even made the severe cycling necessary, as wrestlers with low energy requirements could have had more difficulty controlling weight. They recommended longitudinal studies be conducted to assess any health changes resulting from weight restriction and fluctuation.

Although the body fat for both groups of wrestlers in this study is similar, an increase of fat over lean has been noted during fast weight regain, and a redistribution of fat is suggested as possible. Research is cited that shows increased preference for fat in the diet among weight cycling female rats.

The researchers speculate there may be psychological implications of repeated weight cycling, including frustration over the increasing difficulty in losing weight, which could lead to unhealthy methods of weight loss.

The high school or college wrestler differs from the typical weight cycler in the general population in that he is young, male, physically active, well-muscled, with low body fat. His diet and binge cycle is relatively short, usually lasting about three months a year for perhaps three to six years.

Psychologically, as a successful athlete, he is likely to have high self-esteem and strong social support.

Strong statements against excessive weight loss and the fluid and food deprivation practices often used by wrestlers have been issued by the American College of Sports Medicine and the American Medical Association.[5]

The researchers say weight cycling may account for the observed increase in deaths in these ways:

1. Factors that influence coronary risk (such as cholesterol levels) may change with fluctuating weight and end up worse than before.
2. The amount and distribution of body fat as weight is lost and regained may change. During weight loss, a person loses both fat and lean body mass, but may regain mostly fat. This fat tends to settle in the abdomen, a location linked to increased heart disease risk.
3. People may increasingly prefer high-fat diets when they lose and regain weight. Studies have shown that weight-cycling laboratory animals tend to eat more fat.

In view of their findings, they suggest it may be important to look at public health implications of current weight loss practices. They note that about half of American women and one-fourth of men are dieting at any one time, with many of these efforts unsuccessful. Weight is commonly regained and the cycle repeated.

Kelly Brownell, PhD, a psychologist and weight specialist at Yale University involved in the study, says the harmful effects of weight cycling may be equal to the risks of remaining obese.

"The pressure in this society to be thin at all costs may be exacting a serious toll," Brownell says. The study's findings indicate that weight cycling is "potentially a very serious public health issue" because it affects such large numbers of people.

"It may be equally bad to lose the same five pounds 10 times as to lose 50 pounds and regain it once," he said.

The relative risk of increased risk with weight fluctuation is in the range of 1.25 to 2.00, which is similar to the risk attributed to obesity and to several of the cardiovascular risk factors, say Brownell and Rodin. Thus, determining weight cycling effects is an important question.[6]

The harmful effects of weight cycling may equal the risks of remaining obese.

Harvard alums risk disease by "always" dieting

Men risk heart disease, hypertension and diabetes by 'always' dieting, regardless of their weight, according to the Harvard Alumni studies reported by Steven N. Blair, an epidemiologist at the Cooper Institute for Aerobics Research in Dallas.

"One of the fundamental tenets of the weight loss industry is if you get people to eat less, they'll lose weight. And if they lose weight, they'll be better off. And there is no evidence to support either one," Blair said at the American Heart Association's annual epidemiology meeting in March 1994.

Earlier, Blair reported higher mortality with weight loss among the Harvard alumni. His latest report investigates non-fatal disease in 12,025 men, average age 67. The men who said they were always dieting had a heart disease rate of 23.2 percent, compared to 10.6 for those who "never" dieted. Their rates for hypertension were 38.3 percent, compared with 23.4 percent for the group who never dieted, and for diabetes 14.6 percent, compared with 3 percent.

Among men who dieted part of the time – "often," "sometimes," or "rarely" – the more they dieted, the higher their rates of disease. These findings held true even among the leanest group of men, and were basically unchanged by weight gain, physical activity, smoking or alcohol intake.

In addition to reporting dieting frequency, the men identified their shape variation at six points through life, total pounds lost, and the number of times they had lost 5, 10, 20 and 30 or more pounds.

In view of his findings, Blair advises people to keep a stable weight and avoid either weight gain or weight loss.[7]

Bone loss with weight loss

Several studies of large population bases show higher mortality rates with weight loss, causing researchers to puzzle over the possible mechanisms whereby weight loss could cause longterm harm, even though it seems beneficial in reducing obesity-related risk factors in short-term studies.

One possible mechanism may be the bone mineral loss which accompanies weight loss. Weight cycling may increase this loss.

Mineral content in women's bones diminishes with weight loss, even when adequate nutrition and aerobic exercise are present. These findings from the USDA Human Research Center in Grand Forks, N.D., support clues which may explain recent findings in federal studies of potentially higher mortality with weight loss. The Grand Forks Center tested 14

"It may be equally bad to lose the same five pounds 10 times as to lose 50 pounds and regain it once."

— Kelly Brownell

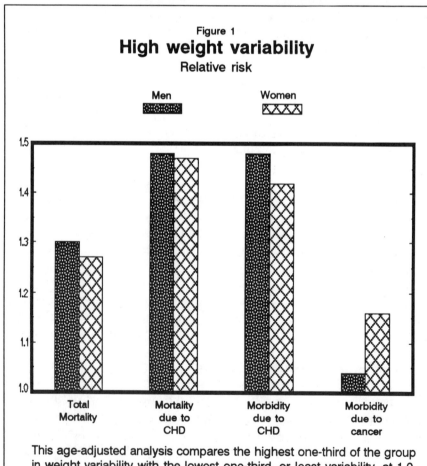

Figure 1
High weight variability
Relative risk

Men

Women

This age-adjusted analysis compares the highest one-third of the group in weight variability with the lowest one-third, or least variability, at 1.0. CHD denotes coronary heart disease. All variables except cancer were significantly higher with weight variability.

HEALTHY WEIGHT JOURNAL(O&H)/LISSNER

women, age 21-38, in a five-month residential program using dual energy x-ray absorptiometry (DXA) to assess bone mineral status and soft tissue composition. The women lost 8.1 kg on a moderate nutrient-adequate diet with an aerobic exercise program. Both bone mineral content and bone mineral density decreased (36 g and .01 g/cm2 respectively).

Similar results were found at the Osteoporosis Research Centre in Copenhagen, Denmark. Using the DXA method, the study reports 51 obese patients averaged a 5.9 percent loss of total body bone mineral/ TBBM during 15 weeks. One patient, who lost 45 kg, lost 754 g bone mineral in nine months. Greater mineral loss was reported in legs than arms. Postmenopausal women who did not get estrogen replacement tended to lose more bone mineral. Bone mineral loss correlated with body fat loss, not with fat-free mass loss, so that as more fat was lost, more mineral was lost as well.

When patients maintained their weight loss, they lost no more bone. If they regained, bone was regained as well. The Danish researchers concluded this level of bone loss was normal for weight loss in obese persons. They suggest an initiating factor in bone loss may be having less weight bearing on the bones.

Hank Lukaski, director of the Grand Forks Center, says people have the potential to regain some bone loss when they regain weight. But it is unknown whether bone mineral content and bone density are fully or only partially restored, or whether bone quality is as good as before, or how essential trace elements are affected. Further, the effect on bone quality of repeated bouts of weight loss and regain are unknown, Lukaski says.[8]

Weight cycling increases stress

People with a history of weight cycling showed greater pathologic characteristics than those with stable weights, independent of weight, in recent research by John Foreyt, PhD, of Baylor College of Medicine, Houston, TX, and colleagues at Yale and the University of Nevada.[9] The researchers suggest that weight cycling may be causal to the mental distress and pathology they found.

Men and women whose weight fluctuated up or down, as little as five pounds in a year, reported lower feelings of well-being, more out-of-control eating, and higher stress levels than people whose weight was stable in this study. And this was true regardless of their body weight.

The researchers say they did not expect such a large number of significant findings with the tight five-pound categories: "Psychologically, such small shifts in weight in both normal weight and obese individuals may be very important."

In obese women, weight maintenance was associated with fewer significant negative life stressors.

Weight fluctuation was strongly associated with negative psychological effects in both normal weight and obese individuals. Weight change and obesity were also associated with a poorer psychological score.

The researchers studied 497 adults, stratified into five age groups, 25 normal weight and 25 obese in each age and sex category.

The subjects were assessed twice with the Brownell Weight Cycling Questionnaire, which measures current dieting, weight satisfaction, abnormal eating patterns and body image. They reported on health, weight

Weight variability in Sweden

Higher mortality with weight cycling is cautiously supported by studies in Sweden. Variability in body weight measured over 17 years was independently related to mortality for 1,462 women, ages 50 to 72 (at last exam). For 855 men, age 75, measured five times in 25 years, results were the same.

Loss of body weight was independently related to mortality for both men and women. Attempts were made to control for disease states.[53]

fluctuation, feelings of well-being and depression, stressful life events, and eating self-efficacy (ability to control urges to overeat in high-risk situations). Their weight was assessed over one year to classify them, through a weight change of 5 pounds or more, as maintainers, gainers or losers.

The researchers suggest that attempts at weight loss may be stressful for various reasons, including the self-denial required, the disruption of routine, and a concern about failure. Repeated failures to control weight may reduce one's feeling of self-efficacy, and add to feelings of depression.

"Once inappropriate dieting is initiated, regardless of body weight, fluctuations and increasing obesity may follow," says their report. They cite research that shows that among obese individuals, more than half fluctuate up or down 12 pounds over intervals of 1 to 5 years.

While the researchers suggest that weight change likely causes these adverse effects, they grant the reverse is possible – psychological distress may cause weight change. They recommend further research on assessing and treating weight fluctuation for individuals of all weights.

Weight cycling apprears consistently linked to increased psychopathology, lower life satisfaction, more disturbed eating in general, and perhaps increased risk for binge eating in the research, Brownell and Rodin report.

They cite research by Everson and Matthews that found lower levels of life satisfaction related to increased weight cycling in women, but not men. A study of a large sample of runners found weight cycling associated with higher levels of disturbed eating practices. Other studies show repeated or chronic dieting may predispose an individual to disordered eating, including binge eating. One study showed restrained eating (dieting) to be a stonger predictor of weight fluctuation than body weight itself.

Weight fluctuation was strongly associated with negative psychological effects in both normal weight and obese individuals.

Findings stir controversy

The recent findings are likely to be controversial and to further fuel the weight cycling debate among scientists, says Claude Bouchard, PhD, of Laval University, Quebec, in an editorial in the same issue of the *New England Journal of Medicine* as the Lissner study.

Bouchard notes that a recent review of 18 studies of weight cycling in rodents, by Hill and Reed, found no clear evidence that weight cycling makes future weight loss harder and weight gain easier.

They found no evidence that weight cycling increases total body fat or central adiposity, increases subsequent caloric intake, increases food efficiency, decreases energy expenditure, or increases blood pressure, insulin resistance, or cholesterol levels. However, Bouchard suggests there may be a preference for dietary fat in refeeding and that the observed risks could result from higher fat intake.

Rat studies may not provide the weight cycling information needed for humans and, given that human studies are difficult to design, this may be why weight cycling studies give such confusing and conflicting results, says Carolyn Berdanier, PhD, a researcher at the University of Georgia.

Berdanier says rats and mice differ from humans in several important ways. Most critically to weight cycling research, they continue to grow in length throughout their lives. This growth is expensive in calories, and affects the degree of body fat storage, keeping them leaner.

Also, food restriction does not work with genetically obese mice and rats. When restricted and kept at a low body weight, they still have the same percent body fat as their larger litter mates, she reports.[10]

In reviewing the literature on human studies, Rena Wing, PhD, University of Pittsburgh School of Medicine, reports the majority of studies do not show negative effects from weight cycling on total body fat, body fat distribution, or resting energy expenditure, and do not support the hypothesis that weight cycling makes subsequent efforts at weight loss more difficult.[11]

In seeking to refute the idea that cycling makes weight loss more difficult, she offers evidence that people may not stick to their diet as well on the second try. Diet adherance for the first cycle is higher than for the second and third cycles in some studies.

However, Wing acknowledges the evidence does suggest that weight cycling may have adverse effects on cardiovascular disease and all-cause mortality.

Wing questions the methodology used in some studies, particularly related to the criteria used to define weight cycling and the inability to control for confounding variables such as involuntary weight loss related to illness.

She points out that a better definition of weight cycling needs to be developed. If it is cycling that appears to influence the risk, then the number of weight changes rather than the magnitude, needs to be emphasized. Instead, a definition which includes large weight changes, such as in the Lissner study, emphasizes these large changes over several smaller changes.

Wing says the concern about weight cycling arose from a concern about dieting and unsuccessful weight loss efforts. Research should return to this hypothesis, she says, and focus on obese individuals who have had numerous voluntary weight cycles. She notes the outcome may be very different in obese than normal weight individuals.

The important question, says Wing, is whether the risks of obesity are greater or less than the risks of attempting to lose weight, succeeding for a period ot time (with the associated improvements in glycemic control, cholesterol, and blood pressure) and then regaining the weight (with a worsening of risk factors). No studies have compared these patterns in the obese population.

Bouchard points out that human populations are not easily investigated, because researchers must obtain measurements over a long period of time, assess many risk factors, and control for numerous variables. It is also difficult to disentangle voluntary weight loss from other causes of weight variability.

An important question in weight fluctuation research is whether weight loss is voluntary, or involuntary and the result of other factors, such as disease or mood disorders, which may lead to increased mortality. Available human studies on large data bases have not determined why weight loss and gain occurred, even though most have tried to control for pre-existing disease, such as cancer, by excluding deaths in the first three to five years.

Even though weight fluctuation appears to be highly correlated with dieting, this cannot be assumed. Scientists are calling for future research to distinguish reasons for weight change.

However, Brownell and Rodin cite two studies which find close relationships. In one, variability was correlated with a history of dieting; in theother, individuals who reported being on a diet at baseline had larger changes in weight over the next 10 years than those not initially dieting.

Clearer definitions, and more accurate ways of measuring weight cycling according to these definitions, need to be developed. Weight cycling research has used a variety of definitions, and applied them to population data bases which were unable to give the information needed. This may be a reason for the inconsistent and controversial results found, say researchers.

Bouchard calls for well-designed animal studies which control for diet composition across the cycles of weight gain and loss, and which measure changes in fat location.

Some studies show fat may be redistributed during weight loss and regain, so that there is a higher percent body fat at the end of a cycle than at the beginning, or more fat is deposited around the waist.

Brownell and Rodin suggest that fat redistribution could be a mechanism whereby weight cycling is related to higher health risks. They cite studies which show a higher degree of waist-hip ratio with weight cycling and with increased number of pregnancies. "Pregnancy may be a form of weight cycling that could affect risk through both weight and body fat distribution," they note.

NIH Task Force stirs controversy

In late 1994, the nine-member NIH National Task Force on the Prevention and Treatment of Obesity published a consensus article in the Journal of the American Medical Association that discounted any harmful effects of weight cycling. It urged obese individuals not to "allow concerns about hazards of weight cycling to deter them," from weight loss efforts.[12]

The controversial article reviewed weight cycling research from 43 articles, and concluded that because many of the findings are not clear or in the same direction, they need not be considered critical for decision-making at this time.

The report noted that most concerns focus on the possibly harmful effects in three major areas:
* psychological well-being,
* morbidity and mortality, and
* metabolism and subsequent weight loss efforts.

However, it mentioned psychological effects only briefly, and discounted the research it reviewed on morbidity and mortality.

The Task Force acknowledged that several large studies have shown increased health risks with weight fluctuation for all-cause and cardiovascular mortality. In some of these, weight variance was associated with increased mortality, even after controlling for heart disease risk factors and preexisting disease that might influence weight. In addition, the report said, weight loss over time has been found to be associated with increased mortality, even when care is taken to exclude smoking and preexisting illness.

But the Task Force faults these studies for unclear definitions of weight cycling and failure to distinguish between voluntary and involuntary weight loss, the possible effects of depression and not identifying any mechanism to explain an adverse effect. And they say that it's not clear

Clearer definitions and more accurate ways of measuring weight cycling need to be developed.

from the studies that weight cycling is related to metabolic changes, percentage or distribution of body fat, or to an increased difficulty in subsequent weight loss attempts.

The Task Force said there is no convincing evidence that weight cycling has adverse effects on body composition, energy expenditure, risk factors for cardiovascular disease, or the effectiveness of future efforts at weight loss. While this statement does not answer concerns about increased morbidity and mortality, the report said this evidence is not sufficiently compelling to override the potential benefits of moderate weight loss in obese patients.

The report does recommend that individuals who are not obese and have no risk factors for obesity-related illness should not attempt weight loss, but instead focus on preventing weight gain with increased physical activity and healthy diet. Obese individuals who undertake weight loss efforts are advised to commit to lifelong changes in their behavioral patterns, diet and physical activity.

Several prominent researchers disagreed with the Task Force conclusions. Foreyt, a Task Force member, said there are "very clear adverse psychological effects" to weight cycling.

Dieting and weight cycling are commonly a part of, and may lead to, the onset of eating disorders, say several eating disorder specialists.

Brownell said dieting and weight cycling have possible negative psychological effects, such as negative body image, depression and an adverse effect on personal relationships.

Further, the Task Force is premature in dismissing the possibility of a long-term metabolic slowdown from weight cycling, Brownell says.

Susan Wooley, PhD, an obesity and eating disorder specialist in Cincinnati, says the medical community should wait to okay widespread dieting and weight cycling until favorable long term results are shown.

She points out the fallacy in Task Force thinking that because weight fluctuation has proven dangerous primarily in studies of people at normal weight, it may therefore be safe for obese persons. "These findings, raising the specter of either pointlessness or harm for both the fat and thin, might equally well be used to disqualify dieting altogether."

Others question whether the Task Force acts as an independent entity. Although a federal NIH advisory group, the Task Force appears to be closely tied to the weight loss industry. "Probably most if not all of the Task Force members have industry funding now, or have had recently," says one source close to the Task Force. *Healthy Weight Journal* has twice requested information on industry funding of Task Force members under the Freedom of Information Act, and has yet to receive the information.

The Task Force continues to focus only on weight loss treatment, even in the face of abysmal failure rates of all treatments, charges Pat Lyons, RN, MA, a regional health educator for Kaiser Permanente in Oakland, Calif. She cites the recent Task Force recommendation to ease state and federal regulations that now restrict the long-term use of obesity drugs.

"The course they are on at present – to advocate weight loss at any cost in a social climate that perpetuates discrimination against fat people – will indeed have high costs for millions of Americans," Lyons said.

The Task Force is slated for reorganization and a possible change in direction soon.

"These findings, raising the specter of either pointlessness or harm for both the fat and thin, might equally well be used to disqualify dieting altogether."
— Susan Wooley

10. Mortality increase with weight loss

Does weight loss escalate the risk of death?

A series of large population studies suggests this area needs further study.

Despite the fact that weight loss brings improvements in health risk factors such as blood pressure, cholesterol and blood glucose, there is considerable evidence that weight loss may increase risk of early mortality instead of decreasing it.

The panel for the March 1992 NIH conference on Methods for Voluntary Weight Loss and Control received a startling answer when it asked the question: "What are the benefits and adverse effects of weight loss?"

Scientists from the Centers for Disease Control and Prevention in Atlanta, and others, informed the panel there is little evidence that weight loss lowers mortality rates. On the contrary, most studies show weight loss in the general population is associated with increased risk of death.[1]

Framingham Heart Study

Men and women who lost weight through 10 years had the highest death rates during 18 years of follow-up in an NIH study based on the Framingham data, reported Millicent Higgins, MD, Associate Director of the Epidemiology and Biometry Program at the National Heart, Lung and Blood Institute, NIH, in Bethesda, Md.

In younger men, death rates were lowest in the weight stable group. In older men death rates were lowest in the weight gain group (which was also lower in weight than the other two).

In younger women, mortality rates were similar in all groups for the first six years; after that they were lowest in the weight gain group. In older women, mortality rates were similar for the weight stable and weight gain groups.

Subjects were measured at two-year intervals for 10 years. Deaths the next four years were excluded. Age and initial weights, but not smoking, were adjusted.

More of the weight loss group were smokers at the final exam, and fewer had quit smoking.

CARDIA

Higgins also reported to the panel on the CARDIA study (Coronary Artery Risk Development in Young Adults). Again, weight loss was associated with increased morbidity and mortality as well as, paradoxically, improvements in blood pressure and lipid factors.

This study included 3,593 young men and women, ages 18 to 30, examined initially, then at two and five years. Three groups were defined by their first two exams: weight stable; weight loss of 5 or more pounds; weight gain of 5 or more pounds. They were subdivided by whether their weight at five years was above or below the median for gain.

Women in the weight loss group were initially heavier and had higher rates of smoking.

There is little evidence that weight loss lowers mortality rates. On the contrary, most studies show weight loss is associated with increased risk of death.

— CDC

Higgins said smoking was associated with leanness and weight loss, and may account in part for these results. More of the weight gain group had quit smoking (nearly 20 percent of women smokers in the weight gain group had quit, compared with about 8 percent in the other two; about 23 percent of men smokers had quit in the weight gain group compared with 4 to 6 percent in the other two).

NHANES I follow-up

The Centers of Disease Control NHANES I Follow-up study, reported by Elsie Pamuk, PhD, epidemiologist at CDC in Atlanta, found weight loss associated with increased risk of death for both men and women, also for cardiovascular and noncardiovascular diseases. The more weight lost, the higher the risk (see Figure 1 and Figure 2, page 82).

Maintaining a stable weight meant no increased risk for moderately overweight men and women (BMI 26 to 29). But a weight loss of 15 percent or more (of maximum weight) was associated with higher death rates, regardless of their weight.

For women in all three weight groups, any amount of weight loss increased their mortality rate. This was true of men, also, except for men in the highest weight group (BMI 29 or higher) for whom a moderate weight loss (between 5 and 15 percent) seemed beneficial. Losing more weight, however, again increased their risk.

This study used NHANES I data of 2,140 men and 2,550 women, age 45 to 74, based on measurements in 1971-75 and their recall of the heaviest weight they had ever been. They were followed for about 10 years (through 1987), with deaths in the first five years excluded. Adjustments were also made for previously diagnosed illness.

Subjects were divided into three groups by their maximum weight, then subdivided into three categories by percent of maximum weight lost. Nearly two-thirds had lost 5 percent or more.

The study was adjusted for age, race, parity for women and baseline smoking.

Numerous analyses were performed to control for pre-existing illness. However, the results still held. They were even intensified, for example, when cardiovascular disease was looked at separately, although it is not apparently related to weight loss.

Similarly, attempts were made to control for smoking by isolating three baseline categories: never smoked, former smoker and current smoker. Analysis is now being performed separately with the never smoked group.

Ten studies consistent

A "surprising consistency" in results from 10 widely varying studies indicates that weight loss is invariably and usually progressively associated with high mortality, reported Reubin Andres, MD, clinical director of the National Institute on Aging Gerontology Research Center, NIH, Baltimore.

The studies varied widely in design, technique, initial "cleanup" for disease and smoking issues, periods of follow-up (8 to 22 years), age of subjects and populations (Figure 3, page 84).

Andres concludes that, while for certain conditions weight loss may be a benefit, "For the general population, the results of the 10 studies do not support the idea that losing weight will increase longevity. . . (but) the

For women in all three weight groups, any amount of weight loss increased their mortality rate.

*Mortality rates
increased from
1.5 to 2.8
for women
at the
highest weight level,
as weight loss
increased from
less than 5 percent to
15 percent or more
of total weight.*

– CDC

Figure 1
Risks of weight loss
NHANES I Follow-up, CDC

Maximum weight lost	Maximum BMI		
Men	**<26**	**26-29**	**29+**
<5%	1.0	0.9	1.5
5-<15%	1.1	1.3	1.2
15%+	1.8	2.1	2.0
Women			
<5%	1.0	0.8	1.5
5-<15%	1.5	1.4	1.8
15%+	2.7	1.9	2.8

CDC study compares effects of weight loss at three weight levels from all causes. Higher mortality is associated with higher weight loss for all levels. The exception is that moderate weight loss appears beneficial in very overweight men.

HEALTHY WEIGHT JOURNAL(O&H)/NIH CONF 1992

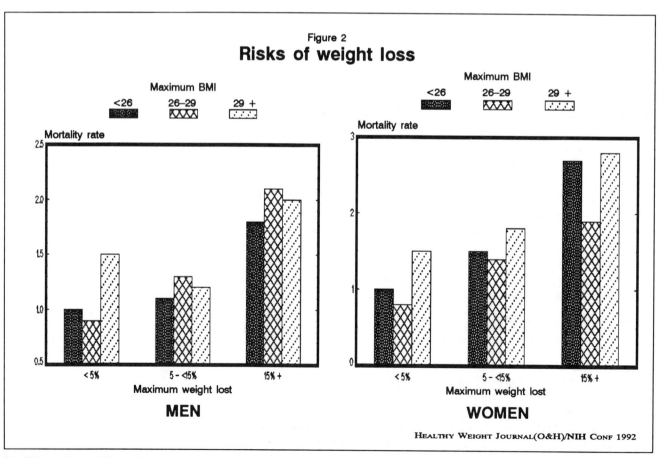

Figure 2
Risks of weight loss

MEN

WOMEN

HEALTHY WEIGHT JOURNAL(O&H)/NIH CONF 1992

opposite conclusion.

"If body weight for optimal survival increases with age, then weight gain with passage of time is permissible and can even be recommended."

MRFIT

Two studies in progress, MRFIT (Multiple Risk Factor Intervention Trial) and the Harvard Alumni Study, suggest higher rates of morbidity and mortality for men with higher levels of weight fluctuation, reported Steven Blair, PED, Director of Epidemiology, Cooper Institute for Aerobics Research, Dallas. In addition to weight cycling effects, he said, MRFIT also shows highest death rates for men who lose weight, lowest risk with stable weight, and slightly elevated risk with weight gain.

The MRFIT prevention study followed for 10 years 10,534 men who were initially in the upper 10 to 15 percent of risk for coronary heart disease, but with no clinical evidence of it. Men with severe obesity (over 1.5 times ideal weight) were excluded, as were deaths in the first year of follow-up. A randomly assigned special intervention group of 5,323 were examined every 4 months; the others had annual exams.

Results show progressively higher mortality for coronary heart disease, cardiovascular disease and all causes: with higher incidence of weight fluctuation; with weight cycling once or more; and with weight loss. With weight gain there was slightly increased risk. In general, the effects were heightened for the special intervention group.

The study is controlled for age, race, cholesterol levels, weight, smoking, alcohol consumption and physical activity and also for changes in smoking, alcohol consumption and physical activity.

MRFIT shows highest death rates for men who lose weight and lowest risk with stable weight.

Harvard alumni

The Harvard Alumni Study findings, given by Blair, are consistent with MRFIT in that men with the highest weight fluctuation had the highest disease rates, and men with the lowest fluctuation the lowest disease rates.

Weight fluctuation in the ongoing study, which began in 1962 and includes 11,140 men, was assessed by two methods in the 1988 questionnaire.

From nine body drawings the men checked those that best matched their shape at present, at college entrance, and at ages 25, 40, 50 and 60. They also reported the number of times they had lost weight (under 5 pounds, 5, 10, 20, and 50 or more pounds) and this was calculated as total lifetime pounds loss.

Defining three groups by degree of weight fluctuation, the Harvard study finds these progressively higher rates of nonfatal diseases with higher weight fluctuation:

a. Coronary heart disease (1.00, 1.15, 1.30)

b. Myocardial infarction (1.00, 1.12, 1.29)

c. Hypertension (1.00, 1.07, 1.11)

d. Diabetes Type II (1.00, 1.09, 1.42)

Defining three categories by total pounds lost, the study finds progressively higher rates of the above conditions with more pounds lost.

Figure 3

Risks of weight loss

Ten studies

	Loss in BMI (adj. to 10 yr)	Relative risk of death	
		Men	Women
Framingham	0 - 2.5	1.40	1.10
	>2.5	1.90	1.80
Dutch Elderly	5+	1.45	1.05
Alameda County	0.5	1.56	
Baltimore Aging	0.4 - 2.8	1.25	
	>2.8	1.33	
Honolulu Heart	>0.4	1.45	
Lipid Research	0.6	1.27	
British Heart	2 - 5	1.60	
	>5	2.00	

Loss of weight is associated with mortality in these studies. Two other studies reporting only gains (Paris Prospective and Harvard Alumni) found highest risk in the lowest gain group. In another study mortality was unrelated to weight loss or gain, Andres.

HEALTHY WEIGHT JOURNAL(O&H)/NIH CONF 1992

Opposing findings

David Williamson, PhD, epidemiologist, Centers for Disease Control, Atlanta, reported studies which showed opposite results, but says these were seriously flawed. A Metropolitan Life Insurance study found that moderately overweight men who reduced weight decreased their mortality rate to 20 percent lower than men who did not reduce; for women the reduction in mortality was 37 percent. In the more severely overweight group, men who lost weight decreased mortality rate 39 percent; women 16 percent.

Findings preliminary

In these studies, which find higher mortality with weight loss, two possibly confounding issues are pre-existing illness and smoking. However, the researchers say they believe these factors would not change the results.

Special analyses were conducted on various factors in attempts to control for the effects of diseases associated with weight loss which could lead to early death. The researchers looked at cardiovascular disease, which is not a wasting disease, separately from other diseases, and found an even stronger relationship. They excluded all deaths for a period of years.

Blair says that he has been examining this effect of higher mortality with weight loss and weight fluctuation for three years, doing "all sorts of analysis – and can't make it go away." He says there appears to be no separate effect with cancer which, as a wasting disease, one might expect.

Furthermore, Blair says, "I do not believe this can be explained by changes in smoking. When we look at smokers, never smokers or intermittent smokers, we don't see any difference. Results are in the same direction."

The NHANES I Follow-up study at CDC is now looking separately at nonsmokers. Pamuk says she doesn't think the results will be much different, because, "the study shows the same effects in older women, and not many were smokers."

Since these findings are preliminary, the NIH panel statement did not recommend treatment changes. It reads, in part:

"While the data are provocative, they are sufficiently inconclusive and should not dictate clinical practice. Specific research efforts addressing this question are urgently needed. The fact that many people who stop smoking gain weight makes comparisons of weight gainers and weight losers more difficult. Also that most of the studies cannot distinguish purposeful weight loss from that associated with illness, psychosocial distress, or other reasons. We need to know much more about the individuals who have lost weight and why they, unlike participants in programs, appear to keep weight off."

The evidence on weight cycling was found similarly controversial: "Data presented on the health effects of repeated weight gains and losses, or weight cycling, also are inconclusive. Cycling appears to affect energy metabolism and may result in faster regains of weight, but the evidence that weight cycling has longer term negative effects on psychological and physical health needs further confirmation."

Pamuk suggests these findings may be showing that losing weight, by itself, does not always improve health, or that some types of voluntary weight loss may be harmful. More attention needs to be paid to how the weight is lost and whether it is sustained, she says.

It is difficult to work with data which was collected for other purposes, as in the NHANES follow-up, she notes. Needed information may not be available. There are "just not enough facts out there," and research money is tight.

However, Pamuk suggests that health recommendations may need to be reconsidered. "The general assumption has been that weight loss is helpful . . . but perhaps maintaining stable weight will be found to be the best course."

From the public health view, Williamson says he feels there should be less focus "on loss of weight, and more on maintaining healthy behaviors, especially for people who are moderately overweight."

Both assert that a primary health objective should be the prevention of obesity, through early establishment of a healthy diet and regular phsycial activity.

Despite these findings, the reports still confirmed an improvement of cardiovascular risk factors with weight loss, and higher mortality was generally associated with obesity.

"The general assumption has been that weight loss is helpful . . . but perhaps maintaining stable weight will be found to be the best course."

— Elsie Pamuk

Voluntary weight loss

In addressing these issues further, Williamson says no credible causal theory has been suggested to explain how weight loss could, in the short run improve risk factors for chronic disease, but in the long run increase mortality.

He questions whether the epidemiologic studies are free of the biases in differentiating between volunatry and involuntary weight loss,

Weight loss may be associated with increase in some unrecognized risk factor for cardiovascular disease.

or failing to identify individuals who may have illnesses causing them to lose weight. Also some studies do not control adequately for smoking.

Williamson reported tentative findings from the Cancer Prevention Study at the North American Association for the Study of Obesity meeting in Atlanta in September 1992, which he says were free of these biases.

The cancer study includes 12-year survival data on 594,551 individuals who were asked whether weight loss was voluntary or involuntary. Smoking history and health status at the time the survey was administered were controlled for.

In most of the groups, voluntary weight loss was either not statistically associated with subsequent mortality, or appeared protective. The strongest protective effect of voluntary weight loss was for women with the poorest health. For healthy older women who had never smoked, weight gain seemed to exert a protective effect.

It is emphasized that these studies are preliminary. More research is needed to continue to analyze possible confounding factors such as pre-existing illness, quitting smoking and other factors. It needs to be determined who the people losing weight are, and why they have increased mortality.[2]

Evidence remains strong

Follow-up studies since the 1992 conference have found little new information to explain the seeming paradoxes of these issues.

In early 1995, Karen Petersmarck, a dietitian and PhD candidate at Michigan State University, reviewed the scientific literature to date and reported that, despite the limitations of each study (most notably the lack of information on lifetime weight history, with weight generally having been measured at only two points in time) the evidence for higher motality with weight loss is strong.[3]

"Each of the studies was conducted by capable researchers. Each involves a large study population, and each controls for known or possible confounders to the extent possible in the data set. The fact that so many of these carefully-done prospective studies suggest the same association between weight loss and increased mortality makes it less likely that the finding was just a fluke or a beta statistical error," she said.

Petersmarck has compiled the following information on possible explanations for increased mortality with weight loss.

How could risk increase with weight loss?

by Karen Petersmarck

How could it be that weight loss improves health risk factors but increases the chance of early mortality? This question has been raised all over the world by ethical researchers, clinicians, policy makers and concerned consumers. Gary Cutter[4] offered the following possible explanations:

1. Perhaps large amounts of weight loss are associated with myocardial or atrophy and/or long-term electrolyte disturbances that leave the heart vulnerable to lethal arrhythmias and/or ischemic problems. However, if this were the explanation, the excess mortality should arise in sudden deaths and this has not been reported except in investigations of deaths from very low calorie diets in the 1970s.[5]

2. A more plausible explanation is that weight loss does confer health benefits, but does not make up for the increased risk that was

incurred while weight was elevated.

3. Perhaps excess weight carried earlier in life may be more detrimental than weight added later in life. If this is true, weight loss in young adults may be more successful in delaying mortality than weight loss in older individuals. Combining young losers with older losers may obscure benefits of weight loss in the younger group. Earlier life weight history would be an important variable to somehow quantify and account for in statistical analysis.

4. It could be that those successful in losing weight were losing it in response to fear about their health brought on by the onset of cardiac symptoms or learning about high blood pressure of high cholesterol. Even in analyses where all individuals with risk factors are grouped together, it would be difficult to control for the degree of risk or the subjects's fear of the consequences of risk. Thus the most successful weight losers may have greater initial risk than those not losing weight. This could explain increased mortality in the "successful" weight loss groups.

5. Perhaps weight loss is a surrogate for some other condition which causes weight loss, such as alcoholism, a poor quality diet (with concomitant reduced immune function), poor control of diabetes, or higher surgical risk.

6. Weight loss over two points in time may be a marker for weight cycling. This idea is supported by the finding of Lee and Paffenbarger (1992) that men who had lost or gained more than 5 kg during the study period also had the highest total amounts of weight loss over their lifetime. It is also supported by the documented fact that 75 to 95 percent of individuals who lose weight regain it.

7. Since advancing age increases risk of death, it is possible that, even in the fact of statistical "adjustment" for age, the effect of increasing mortality is not fully accounted for with the statistical control among the groups.

Some other ideas about causation have been suggested by others:

8. Weight loss may be associated with increase in some unrecognized risk factor for cardiovascular disease, such as elevated concentrations of arachidonic acid and low levels of omega-3 fatty acid reserves.[6, 7]

9. Along the same line of thought, Adelle Davis, a popular nutrition writer in the 1950s, cautioned against extreme weight loss because environmental pollutants that are potentially cancer-promoting or cardiotoxic such as DDT are stored in fat, and could be increased in concentration in the blood when fat stores are mobilized.

10. Weight loss may be associated with some demineralization of bones, thus increasing the incidence of osteoporosis in older women. Osteporosis is sometimes called "the silent killer," because it leads to hip fractures in older women which precipitate a chain of events leading to death within a few months of the facture.[8]

11. It may be that the weight that is regained after dieting is preferentially deposited in abdominal visceral fat stores. People with high abdominal visceral fat stores are generally acknowledged to be at higher risk of heart disease. This hypothesis is not supported by

Weight regained after dieting may be preferentially deposited in abdominal visceral fat stores.

human studies of weight gain,[9, 10] or by the bulk of animal research,[11] but cannot be ruled out at this time.

12. It is known that weight loss improves cholesterol concentrations and blood pressure, while weight gain worsens these risk factors. Perhaps the rate of worsening with weight regain is faster than the rate of improvement with weight loss. If this were true, an individual who lost weight and then regained it could end up with a higher cholesterol concentration or blood pressure than he had before losing the weight. There are no published large-sclae studies, to date, that address this question.

11. Thinness: a cultural obsession

At no time in history have the pressures to be thin been more severe than now.

This pressure, and the severe oppression of large people in our society, is driving many women into a life of chronic dieting – no matter what the cost may be to their health. They are willing to do almost anything to lose weight. At this moment, an estimated 40 percent of American women are trying to lose weight, even though many of them are not overweight.

Thin obsession is creating a crisis that is shattering the lives of women, children and their families. Yet it is a crisis that is not widely recognized or being dealt with effectively.

Weight obsession is strongly linked to a growing "epidemic" of eating disorders which severely limit the potential for women of all weights, and increasingly men as well. It also increases the prejudice and stigma against which many large people struggle, in education, employment and health care.

"How easily weight obsession is dismissed as an inevitable phase of female development," charges Susan Wooley, PhD, professor of psychology at the University of Cincinnati. "Would things be different if our hospitals and clinics were filled with young men whose educations and careers were arrested by the onset of anorexia nervosa, bulimia, or the need to make dieting and body shaping a full-time pursuit?"

Some experts are calling it a crime against our children, a monster.

"The public conscience is fast asleep," says Naomi Wolf, author of *The Beauty Myth*. The public is silent when young women die, she adds.

This raises a number of questions that need investigation.[1]

How can this happen at a time when women have more freedom and independence than ever before? Who is pressuring women to be abnormally thin (and to a lesser extent, men), and why? And, most critically: How does this pressure affect women of different sizes? How does it affect young girls and children? How does it affect women with eating disorders? What about men?

How does it impact the larger society, community spirit, and the volunteer structure of this nation?

How thin is thin enough?

Some experts are saying the ideal female body type is now at the thinnest 5 percent of a normal weight distribution. This excludes 95 percent of American women, says Jean Kilbourne, EdD, author of *Still Killing Us Softly: Advertising and the Obsession with Thinness*. A "statistical deviation" has been made to seem the norm, with millions of women believing they are abnormal or "too fat." This mass delusion causes enormous suffering for women and becomes a prison for many, even though it sells a lot of products, she charges.[2]

"For women to stay at the official extreme of the weight spectrum requires 95 percent of us to infantilize or rigidify to some degree our mental lives." says Wolf,

Thin obsession is creating a crisis that is shattering the lives of women, children and their families.

Fashions in the female figure

by Beatrice Robinson

Thinness has not always been viewed with such universal fervor and longing (as currently). In earlier times the more voluptuous, abundant female figure was seen as the ideal.

Western taste has idealized three types of women since about 1500.

The first was tummy-centered and often quite fat. W. Bennet and J. Gurin call her the "reproductive figure" in *The Dieter's Dilemma*.

Somewhere around 1650-1700, taste changed throughout Europe to a new ideal which was plump and all bosom and bottom; her narrow waist was designed to emphasize these ample endowments. Bennet and Gurin label this type the "maternal figure".

Then, rather rapidly between 1910 and 1920, this full-blown female figure lost its favor within Anglo-American culture and was replaced by a tubular, lean and slender figure with little remnant of the promising reproductive tummy and with minimal breasts and buttocks. Bennet and Gurin call this the "sexual free agent".

During the 1900s this idealized female form fluctuated, but has become increasingly thinner over the past two to three decades. Over the period from 1959-1978 Playmates in *Playboy* centerfolds dropped from 91 percent of average (for age, height and sex to 84 percent. Similarly, Miss American contestants dropped from 88 percent of normal in the 1960s to 85 percent in the 1970s.

This increasingly thin ideal has created a self-image problem for American women, approximately 75 percent of whom believe they are "too fat." It is partially responsible for the growth in bulimic and anorexic clients that mental-health professionals are increasingly seeing. But one of the most affected groups appear, for the most part, to be suffering in silence: the women who are overweight by health and fashion standards.[s1]

"In less than two decades the acceptable female body size has been whittled down by one-third," report Susan Wooley, Patricia Fallon and Melanie Katzman, editors of *Feminist Perspectives on Eating Disorders,* a book that relates the anguish of eating disorders to the problems of ordinary women and is shaking the foundations of the eating disorder field. They charge that our society demands women give up nourishment and a large share of their bodies.

Increasing pressures on women to be thin are vividly illustrated by a 30-year survey of Miss America contestants and Playboy magazine centerfold girls from 1959 to 1988.

Both of these cultural icons have become thinner and thinner, year by year, and are now at anorexic levels of 13 to 19 percent below their expected weight. (A clinical criteria for anorexia nervosa is 15 percent or more below expected weight.) Miss America entries today have thinner hips than ever before, but Playboy centerfold girls are even thinner. For both, the drop in weight has leveled off, likely because to drop weight further is to risk death by starvation, say the researchers.[3]

Roberta Seid, PhD, University of Southern California, says, "Each era has exacted its own price for beauty, though our era is unique in producing a standard based exclusively on the bare bones of being, which can be disastrous for human health, happiness and productivity,"

In the past, excesses of fashion were severely criticized by social authorities, including doctors, teachers, clergy, parents and feminists, and moralists stressed there were values more important than outward appearance, she says. But "in the late 20th century all these authorities, especially physicians, seemed to agree that one could never be too thin."

Gaunt idols

The pressure by the media to be thin is stronger now than at any time in the last 19 years, according to a recent study that compiled statistics for television commercials on diet foods, diet program foods and chemically based reducing aids, using advertising data from the *Network Television Books.*[4]

The diet-promoting ads increased to over 4.5 percent of all television advertising by 1991, up from almost none in 1973. Of these, most ads are for diet foods.

This is an increasing trend that does not appear to be leveling off, the researchers say.

Is the look for the latter half of the 1990s thinner than ever? Yes, claims a *Newsweek* fashion article: "It is a slimmer, more dissipated vision. . . reedy, boyish women with hollow curves and sinewy lines. . . small, frail-looking. . . wan and disengaged. . . austere as the times. . . human coat hangers. . . Clothes fall off them."[5]

The article says these images have toppled the "curvaceous supermodels" of the past decade.

Newsweek calls this a "return to reality. . . down to earth." Inexplicably the magazine concludes this proves that "men and their appetites" don't rule the world.

'Steeples of bones'

Present-day 'beauties' are women with faces gaunt and angular, necks resembling steeples of bones, as described by Seid. Their arms and legs are unfleshed, full of sharp angles, gangly and disproportionately long.

"Indeed the lean body looks as repressed and controlled as the spirit that must have gotten it that way. . . it offers no softness, no warmth, no tenderness, no mysteries," she writes.

Seid wonders if future historians might think we Americans had fallen in love with death, or if a terror of nuclear destruction had made "fashion play with cadavers and turn them into images of beauty."

The emphasis on dieting is expanding into a new focus on fitness and body sculpting. The thinness craze is lucrative for the fitness industry, and its advertisers are exploiting it heavily.

They are promoting the new body-shaping goal for women as getting thin, lean and hard, but not developing muscles or strength.

The current ideal of female beauty is "anorexics with barbells," Seid notes.

"The fitness craze co-opts the whole idea of power for women, reducing it to narcissism . . . A woman who lifts weights and is also starving herself will have significantly decreased energy and power. Thus, in the guise of offering health, fitness, and expanded opportunities to women, the culture restricts all of these things," says Kilbourne.

Advertising kills softly

Kilbourne argues that the $130 billion advertising industry is powerful as an educational force in America. The cumulative impact of the 1,500 ads the average American is exposed to every day, and the year and a half of life spent watching TV commercials, is overpowering in enforcing thin ideals, she points out.

"The tyranny of the ideal image makes almost all of us feel inferior," Kilbourne says. "We are taught to hate our bodies, and thus learn to hate ourselves. This self-hatred takes an enormous toll. . . (in) feelings of inferiority, anxiety, insecurity, and depression."

And ironically, as they enforce rigid stereotypes, Kilbourne says that advertisers claim to offer women a new 'freedom' through dieting.

An example is a Wendy's restaurant commercial featuring a very thin young woman who announces, "I have a license to eat."

Kilbourne is outraged. "As if eating for women were a privilege rather than a need. Wendy's salad bar and lighter fare have given her freedom to eat."

Young girls in advertising are often shown as vulnerable and sexually alluring. Often females are doing nothing at all in ads but displaying themselves, while males reinforce ownership of them by towering over or grasping them, says Esther Rothblum, PhD, professor of psychology at the University of Vermont.[6]

Advertising tells us we must constantly perfect and change ourselves, says Kilbourne. Advertising urges women to work for self-improvement rather than societal change, to reshape their bodies rather than encourage a more tolerant society.

The media in three ways creates a distorted picture of reality which adversely affects girls and women, says Karin Jasper, PhD, of the Women's Center in Toronto.[7] She says the false messages contribute to the prevalence of eating disorders.

In portraying women, food and weight issues, the media distorts

Present-day 'beauties' are women with faces gaunt and angular, necks resembling steeples of bones.
— Roberta Seid

reality by (1) frequently propagating myths and falsehoods, (2) normalizing or even glamorizing what is abnormal or unhealthy, and (3) creating a false impression of homogeneity by failing to represent whole segments of the real world.

Trouble ahead for kids

These media pressures apear to have severely adverse effects on children and adolescent girls.

Emaciated, vulnerable, passive, childlike females are idealized as their role models. Diet Sprite marketers thought they had this ideal just right recently when they depicted a bony girl listlessly nursing her diet drink, and boasted in the advertisement that she was nicknamed "Skeleton."

A related issue is the potential for promoting child sexual abuse, often linked to eating disorders, in the sexual poses of child models. Calvin Klein perfume ads feature thin, vulnerable, young models in sexually provocative poses, spurring anger among parents of youngsters with eating disorders.

"There's something very sick going on here," said the mother of an anorexic daughter in a Boston consumers group that boycotted the Diet Sprite ad.

Teachers and parents' groups are becoming more and more concerned as they observe disordered eating affecting a younger group of children each year. Kindergartners worry they're too fat; nine-year-old girls have full blown eating disorders; as many as 80 percent of 10-to 11-year-old girls are afflicted with disordered eating.

Fear of fatness, restricted eating and binge eating are so common among girls by age 10, that this may be viewed, in a sense, as a norm for middle-class, preadolescent girls, says a California study.[8]

The study of 494 girls, age 9 to 18 (66 percent white, 23 percent Asian, 4 percent each black and Hispanic) found disordered eating behavior among 30 to 46 percent of 9-year-olds, and 46 to 81 percent of 10-year-olds, increasing progressively with age. Purging was highest at age 15 (11 percent).

Preventive education for eating disorders needs to begin in the primary grades, the California researchers recommended.

Another study in South Carolina found children as young as age 9 with severe eating disorders, including anorexia nervosa and bulimia nervosa. In their study of 5th graders, University of South Carolina medical researchers found over 40 percent felt too fat or wanted to lose weight, even though 80 percent were not overweight. The researchers suggest this bodes trouble ahead.[9]

The shrinking Olympic gymnast

Even female Olympic gymnasts are becoming younger, smaller and much thinner.[10]

Judges now favor children who weigh under 90 pounds as the ideal female gymnasts. Height of those who win has dropped to 4 feet, 10 inches or less, and top female gymnasts maintain body fat levels of under 10 percent. In the past 30 years, average age has dropped from 18 to 16 years. What happened to Olympic traditions of showcasing the world's top athletes in their prime?

"The public is silent when young women die."
— Naomi Wolf

Hearty, nurturing fat
by Angela Barron McBride

I have wanted to become lean, understated, self-contained, abstemious and delicate but continue to value highly being effusive, lavish, emotional, unconstrained and hearty... part of me regards fat as something very positive. It means being nurturing, warm, lavish, hearty, and a host of other praiseworthy qualities.

A large person may be viewed as superior, healthy, generous, profound, towering, powerful, remarkable, eminent. On the other hand, the phrase "bigger is better" has come to be associated with being wasteful, selfish, clumsy, outrageous, angry at our . . . society which no longer particularly values heartiness, generosity and nurturance.[52]

The girls exchange stunted growth and a likely eating disorder for the privilege of competing as Olympic gymnasts, charges the American Anorexia Bulimia Association. The group calls for competition within age and weight categories, and for promoting an appreciation of the aesthetics of grace and maturity in the sport.

The stereotyping of little girls and boys in the media has perhaps never been worse than it is today, says Kilbourne. "Television programs for children are filled with active boys and passive girls, brought to them by commercials for action products for boys and beauty products and dolls for girls."

She says adolescents are especially vulnerable, "given the ominous peer pressure on young people."

Body image issues are severe for adolescent girls today. In a difficult choice, society prescribes for them extreme thinness and, at the same time, high career aspirations. Focusing on one may cancel out the other. Most girls try to comply with both, to sometimes tragic results.

Living as though their bodies were being constantly watched, is a way girls learn to feel disconnected from their bodies, as if they are disembodied, observing themselves from the outside, say these experts.

"Girls do not simply live in their bodies but become aware of how their bodies appear in the eyes of boys . . . By seeing their own bodies as images in boy's eyes, they begin to observe rather than to experience their own bodies; their bodies become "Other" to themselves," say Deborah Tolman, EdD, and Elizabeth Debold, MEd, of Harvard University.[11]

Fat oppression

The oppression of large people helps drive the need to diet and lose weight. Studies show discrimination in hiring and promotion opportunities, in education, in life insurance, in everyday social relationships, and in health care.

The words "do no harm" are fundamental to medical care, but for large people this credo is often ignored. The emphasis on thinness affects the way large people are treated in health care.

Millions of healthy large people are denied health insurance solely because of their weight. Size-acceptance activists say those who seek care may encounter insults, humiliation, or verbal abuse from physicians.

"When a physician, who is expected to provide expertise and offer comfort, offers criticism instead, it can be emotionally devastating – even life threatening," said Pat Lyons and Debora Burgard, health care providers in California, writing in *Feminist Perspectives on Eating Disorders*. "An attitude of 'Lose 50 pounds and call me in the morning' often substitutes for a sound treatment plan. Whether they are seeking care for pink eye, a sprained ankle, a stiff neck, or a gynecological problem, fat women receive weight loss lectures.

"One woman told us that she went to get glasses and was admonished for her weight! This kind of experience would be laughable if it weren't for the tragic consequences that can occur when fat people avoid or delay obtaining needed medical care."[12]

Lyons and Burgard say another woman who had recently had a mastectomy refused to undergo routine Pap smears, despite her apparent risk for cancer, because she had been so humiliated by a physician

"We are taught to hate our bodies, and thus learn to hate ourselves. This self-hatred takes an enormous toll."
— Jean Kilbourne

who said she was too fat for a proper exam.

Even large tumors have been passed over by intolerant doctors.

"A physician told us of a 60-pound abdominal tumor that was overlooked because the thought of palpating a very fat abdomen was abhorrent to the examining physician," they said.

Many women delay or avoid needed health care because they are overweight and fear being criticized or embarrassed, even when they are health care providers themselves and understand the risks they may be taking, reports a Wisconsin study.

In the study, 310 female nurses, nursing assistants, health unit coordinators, and general psychiatric assistants employed at the community hospital were surveyed.

Women in the two groups of large-size women were more likely to report delaying medical care because of embarrassment about weight or because they did not want a lecture regarding their obesity. In the largest group (body mass index of 35 or more) 55 percent said they delayed or canceled doctor appointments because they knew they would be weighed. Another 3 percent did not delay or cancel appointments but refused to be weighed at their visit. About 20 percent of women in the two larger groups said they delayed medical care until they lost weight, compared with only 5 percent of other women. The researchers say there is obviously considerable emotion generated by this topic, "We must work to remove the barriers that keep obese patients out of their physician's offices."[13]

Sally Smith, executive director of the National Association to Advance Fat Acceptance, has a suggestion: "If physicians were to acknowledge that dietary and behavioral treatments for obesity are ineffective, thus shifting the goal from thinness to the goal of health, I believe women would not delay medical care. Fat women deserve no less."

'Good women' keep dieting

Dieting is being called a kind of religion, subscribed to by "good women."

"Certainly these days, when I hear people talking about temptation and sin, guilt and shame, I know they're referring to food rather than sex," Carol Sternhell wrote in Ms. magazine in April 1985. "Everything, for women, boils down to body size."[14]

It is a need to feel empowered that drives women of all ages and backgrounds to continue to diet and judge their bodies harshly despite an awareness of the ill effects of dieting, says Judith Ruskay Rabinor, a New York eating disorder specialist. "Most women focus on dieting and improving their appearance in order to feel powerful in a world that denies them true power."

Wolf says *dieting* is a trivializing word for what is in fact self-inflicted semistarvation. "Hunger makes women feel poor and think poor. Hunger makes successful women feel like failures. . . (The anorexic) is weak, sexless, and voiceless, and can only with difficulty focus on a world beyond her plate. The woman has been killed off in her. She is almost not there."

For large persons, dieting causes problems that did not exist before the diet, size-acceptance leaders charge. They call dieting a destructive practice.

The current ideal of female beauty is "anorexics with barbells."
— Roberta Seid

Dieting encourages "all-or-nothing," "feast or famine" behavior, say Lyons and Burgard. Some foods are "acceptable/legal/healthy" and others are "bad/forbidden/dangerous." And the dieter is "good" or "bad," depending on how she's eating.

"She often feels that she cannot trust her body to regulate itsclf when it comes to food, or even that her body has betrayed her. . . Dieting teaches the dieter to disregard her body's hunger and satiety cues, and instead to make eating decisions based on the diet's prescriptions. . . The ideology of any diet thus reinforces the split between the dieter's mind and her body, and asks her to distrust her body, which is seen as the source of sabotage."

Yet dieting can be hard to give up. They point out that to give up dieting is to give up long-held fantasies of being thin, the dream of being in control over one's body.

Lyons and Burgard say that for large women the desire for such control may stem from wanting to be less vulnerable to being shamed and humiliated about being fat. In addition, women who internalize the oppression and feel their bodies are to blame may wish to punish the bodies they feel have betrayed them.

"Dieting can be very reinforcing, because in the short run, when effort and enthusiasm are the highest, it does result in weight loss. Many dieters also feel they will be better accepted if they are trying to lose weight. The misconception that people are fat because they are lazy, greedy, or the like requires fat people to appear to be actively making the effort to be thin."

Is it about women's freedom?

Why is this gaunt stereotype so persistently promoted and the diversity of real women ignored?

From a feminist perspective, the selling of thinness is seen as a manipulative tool to prevent women from gaining power in the work force.

This travesty is not being perpetuated on women by individual men – who after all have female friends, lovers, wives, sisters, daughters – but by the political power structure and multinational corporations bent on shaping women into the ultimate consumers, perennially dissatisfied with their appearance, says Wolf.

In a searing account, Wolf charges that this power structure, acting largely through the media, especially women's magazines and their advertisers, unite to force women into a competition of continual striving for thinness and beauty. It's a cruel struggle they can't win.

In this struggle, every woman is made to feel a failure in her attempts to perfect her body and face. No matter what her successes in other areas of life, she falls short. Further, she feels that her body is constantly on display and being judged unfavorably.

Wolf also points out that the adverse effects of self-starvation, in the quest for a thin body, keeps women weak, preoccupied, passive, and off track from career ambitions. A 1984 survey by Glamour magazine found respondents most desired goal was not success in work or love, but losing 10 to 15 pounds.

The thinness obsession is seen by many as a way of curbing women's freedom.

Thin mania turns up the pressure

Six women's magazines, *Playboy* magazine and the Miss America contest all have increased their pressures for female thinness over the past 30 years.

Research at American University, Washington, DC, has built on an earlier study of Miss America entries and Playboy centerfold girls which showed a consistent decrease in body size and weight during the 20 years between 1959 and 1978.

The new study finds Miss America contestants continued to decrease in weight between 1979 and 1988. Playboy centerfolds remain extremely thin.

Over the 10-year period, 69 percent of Playboy centerfolds and 60 percent of Miss America contestants were below their expected weight by 15 percent or more. (This is a major criteria for anorexia nervosa.) No differences were found between Miss America winners and contestants.

The researchers find a leveling off at 13 to 19 percent below expected weight. They suggest this has occurred because it is almost impossible to safely go lower.

Compared with 1959 to 1978, Miss America contestants today have proportionately smaller hips. Today's Playboy centerfold is thinner than Miss America entries.

Six women's magazines studied have dramatically increased their emphasis on weight reduction over the 30 years with many more articles on weight loss diets, diet with exercise, and exercise.

The researchers find a new trend of emphasizing exercise, and warn that excessive exercise is a method of purging after binge episodes, often used by eating disordered patients.

They suggest the extreme and increasing pressure for thinness may offer insight into the "epidemic rise" in eating disorders. [83]

Fighting for acceptance in the fitness world

by Pat Lyons, RN, MA, and Debby Burgard, PhD

"Such a pretty face –"

There are few things more insulting than having a relative, friend or, amazingly enough, a total stranger hand you a diet book or article about weight loss, professing concern for your health as justification for rudeness. Sometimes they slip in the phrase, "You have such a pretty face . . ." allowing our imagination to infer how ugly they think our body is. They try to shame us into "caring about ourselves."

Fat people are barraged by contradictory advice from all sides, some of it from "experts," some from friends, relatives and even strangers, and some from out-and-out crackpots. . . And most Americans have been convinced that anything less than total success means shameful failure.

A vigorous and diligent participant in a jogging class described her elation after two years attending the class: "I feel great! My blood pressure came down so I don't have to take my medicine anymore. I'm full of more energy at 53 than ever before, and I just love to come to these classes because we have such a good time." Then she hung her head in obvious sadness, even shame. "I haven't lost any weight, though. I eat a good, nutritious diet and don't have any traces of high blood sugar anymore, but I still weigh about the same as when I started. I don't know what I'm doing wrong."

How has our society's distorted view of success convinced this vigorous, enchanting human being that ultimately, despite all of the improvements she could see in her health, she had failed? That she should agonize one moment is a disgraceful example of how societal attitudes have undermined her self-respect.

There is probably not a fat woman alive who has not experienced a rush of fear while wondering what others will think, do, or say to her when she goes walking or to an exercise or dance class. This fear probably keeps more large women inactive than any other factor, even the fear of injury . . The emotional pain, shame, and humiliation that most of us fat women must endure as a regular, ongoing part of our lives is very real and cannot be ignored or trivialized. Thinner people accuse us of exaggerating, but we are not

> **‘How has our society's distorted view of success convinced this vigorous, enchanting human being that ultimately, she had failed?’**

exaggerating. We can never hope to get beyond this fear, however, unless we face it directly.

One woman tells the story of summoning up her courage to start swimming regularly, going to a local pool. In the locker room, before she had a chance to get in the pool, an angry woman came to her, shaking her fist and hissing: "You should be ashamed of yourself. How dare you show yourself in public the way you look. You're disgusting."

There are ways of preparing for these incidents in advance, dealing with them on the spot, and surviving them afterwards. One thing you must not do is to accept abuse silently and give a home to the feelings of anger, sadness and shame that fester within and immobilize you . . .

You can be witty, you can terrify someone by hurling abuse in return, you can be dignified and aloof and ignore the creep, or you can tell him or her to go to hell. It's up to you. But whatever you do, be sure to get the incident off your chest after it has occurred. Don't brood over it.

Call a friend . . . and tell her or him every last detail, even the parts that shamed or embarrassed you the most. A friend can remind you that you have every right to your anger, sadness or any other feeling. If you can't reach a friend, write (about) it. Get it out of your system. Then, as soon as possible, do something good for yourself - treat yourself to a warm bath, a massage, a good movie; buy yourself flowers or play with a child who loves you. Do not buy into the idea that anyone has a right to try to shame you, that somehow you "deserved" mistreatment because you are fat. No one ever deserves mistreatment.

We have a right to take up space, live fully in our bodies and fully in our lives. By dealing with our feelings honestly and supporting one another in this right, we make it easier for ourselves and for those who will follow in our footsteps.

If our daughters are going to be able to live active lives, we must blaze a trail for them.[15]

Reprinted with permission from Great Shape: The First Fitness Guide for Large Women, by Pat Lyons and Debby Burgard. Copyright 1988.

Naomi Wolf says dieting and thinness began to be female preoccupations when women got the vote around 1920. Never before had there been idealized "the look of sickness, the look of poverty, and the look of nervous exhaustion."

The new, leaner form replaced the more curvaceous one with startling rapidity, Wolf says. It was a great weight shift that must be understood as one of the major historical developments of the century. It was a direct solution to the dangers posed by the women's movement and by economic and reproductive freedom.

"Prolonged and periodic caloric restriction is a means to take the teeth out of this revolution. . . so that women just reaching for power would become weak, preoccupied, and mentally ill in useful ways and in astonishing proportions," said Wolf.

A cultural fixation on female thinness is not an obsession about female beauty but an obsession about female obedience, Wolf charges. It's "about how much social freedom women are going to get away with or concede." Girls are still being admonished to keep their place, not to strive too hard to compete.

The "good girl" today is the thin girl, the one who keeps her appetite for food (and for power, sex and equality) under control, says Jean Kilbourne, of Wellesley College.

"Both men and women are conditioned and socialized to feel that women must be controlled, kept in their place. Women, of course, internalize these messages, said Kilbourne. "Ironically, what is considered sexy today is a look that almost totally suppresses female secondary sexual characteristics, such as large breasts and hips. Thinness is related to decreased fertility and sexuality in women."

Even though there is new sexual freedom for women, it seems that women's bodies are "as terrifying and repulsive as ever, as greatly in need of purification and mortification," says Sternhell.

Kilbourne argues that women are allowed success in the work place if they focus on being thin, maintain a fragile, waifish image, and do not take up too much space. "The pursuit of thinness is a way to compete without threatening men."

Woman as object

The woman-as-object theme – wherein women are seen in the media, Hollywood and Madison Avenue as decorative objects to be viewed, judged, and admired or dismissed – is analyzed by Susan Kano, author of *Making Peace with Food*. Women are dehumanized, she writes, by beauty contests, body-building contests and pornography, as well as by advertisers and the fashion industry, all of which show women as thin mannequins. Women's clothing, which is often tight and has an ornamental purpose with little regard for comfort or ability to move, is part of this.

Rothblum cites research that suggests a man's status depends more on having attractive female partners than on his own physical attractiveness.

Another explanation for pressures to be thin is that as women have moved into previously male-dominated activities, the "traditional" female body shape has developed negative connotations, while the masculine shape has come to symbolize self-discipline and competency.[16]

Negative sterotypes are widely associated with being overweight,

Fat kills
by Betty Rose Dudley

Because of a persistent cough, I sought out a new doctor. After a series of referrals, I ended up with this very young, very thin female doctor, obviously a jogger by the way she dressed.

At first it seemed as if this might be okay. (But) when the exam was finished, she said to me, with a smile, "Well, what are we going to do about you losing weight?"

"We're not going to do anything," I said. "I'm here because I can't get rid of this cough."

She smiled, shook her head, and ordered X-rays and tests.

I thought, "Okay, fair enough."

The next time I saw her she gave me a handful of weight-loss pamphlets, everything from Weight Watchers and Nutri-System to plain old calorie counting.

She said to me, "You should pick one. They're all pretty good."

"I told you, I don't intend to lose weight," I said. "I'm here because of a cough."

"Don't you know that fat kills?"

"I don't believe that. And I don't believe these diets work.."

"If you're depressed I can refer you to psychiatry," she said.

"No thank you. Just tell me about the X-rays," I said.

"Oh, the X-rays!" she said. "We have found an abnormality on your lung. It could be one of many things, including cancer."

I went back for more test results. The woman walked into the room with even more weight-loss pamphlets.

I said, "I have told you many times I'm not interested in dieting."

She threw the pamphlets down, put her hands on her hips, and looked at me with disgust.

"Well, I just don't even know why you bother to come here if you're not going to listen to what I say," she said.

"I came to find out if I have lung cancer," I said through clenched teeth.

"Oh," she said. You could tell she had forgotten.

I did not have lung cancer.
Reprinted from Fat!So?[84]

Slimness: the new religion?

by Susie Orbach

Women come in all shapes and sizes. But the extraordinary variety that is woman's body is systematically ignored in our culture. The richness of our different shapes is reduced to the overriding image of slimness. Models with anorectic bodies display clothes designed to make women into objects, and shop mannequins are literally shaved down each year.

Meanwhile women, not surprisingly, feel "oversized," too big in one part of their body or another, dissatisfied with particular features of their whole body as a "package." Bombarded by images of increasing slimness, women struggle to mirror the new image churned out seasonally.

Even women who have grown up with a reasonably healthy respect for their bodies (hard as this is to do in our culture) and who have not been previously preoccupied with body image are so assaulted with articles, advertisements, diet columns and advice on beauty matters that peddle thinness as a life solution that they find their confidence undermined.

> *The beauty and variety of the female form are judged unacceptable, and instead slimness is promoted for profit and control.*

What was "acceptable" even ten years ago is now outsize. The Western obsession with slimness pushes women into a relentless struggle to press their bodies into smaller and smaller sizes. The beauty and variety of the female form are judged unacceptable, and instead slimness is promoted for profit and control.

As women are encouraged to become smaller and smaller, and the Western obsession intensifies, more and more books are rushed into the marketplace offering new, permanent weight-reduction schemes or advice on how to dress slim, minimize "bad points" and project the perfect body.

Slimness has developed a life of its own. Success, beauty, wealthy, love, sexuality and happiness are promoted as attached to and depending on slimness. Slimness instantly conveys these qualities as through they automatically go together.

Selling body insecurity to women (and increasingly to men too) is a vicious phenomenon. Many a woman has described the solution to an unfortunate encounter, a lousy day with the kids, a low exam result, in terms of "if only I were slim" or "I'm going to lose weight this week."

Because of the pressure to be slim, many women who may not have had a history of eating problems in childhood or adolescence find themselves unwittingly interfering with the self-regulatory system that lets them know what, when and how much to eat.

There is always a new diet to try, always the possibility that this one will bring the accompaniments of happiness, success, love and health. But the schemes fail. Diets turn "normal eaters" into people who are afraid of food. Food takes on all the punishing and magical qualities that anguish the compulsive eater.

This thin obsession that is inflicted on so many women makes it hard to resist the pressure to conform. Rebellion brings with it feelings of uneasiness and freakishness.

It becomes quite difficult even to raise the question of why the massive variety that is woman's shape is systematically degraded; what is so awful and threatening about women's bodies at any size; why isn't fat considered attractive; why stature and fullness are devalued.

Is the stigma that attaches to large or fat women not just another subtle way to divide one woman from another, thus promoting a false and individual solution to what should be at root a social concern – namely, the position of women in our society? Perhaps we can understand the impetus and energy behind the thinness campaign inflicted on so many women as a (possibly unconscious) skewed reaction to women's desires to be regarded seriously and take up more space.

Women look at each other and marvel at how older women manage to achieve *the look, the face, the body* that gives them a place and an acceptability in the world. The driven, induced need to be slim diverts us from concerns that are more truly central to our experience of life. It absorbs an energy that could help us change the world, not just our bodies.

A few brave women in western Europe and the United States are now battling against the prevailing standards, challenging them, turning them upside down, demanding rights for women of all shapes and sizes, classes and colors. But it is an uphill struggle punctured at every point by the hidden (and not so hidden) persuaders, reminding us that slimness is essential and that women must not occupy more than a little space.[18]

Reprinted with permission from Fat Is A Feminist Issue II, by Susie Orbach. Copyright 1982.

particularly for women. The prejudice and discrimination that comes from weightism, or fatism, is well documented in employment, education, medical care and social relationships.[17]

But most feminist leaders are not interested in fat oppression issues.

"Why haven't feminists focused on hatred of fat in our society?" asks Rothblum. Obesity is highly stigmatized even in feminist groups, she says. Tolerance of size is not an issue these groups have embraced, as each woman struggles alone with her weight issues, her appearance, her place as a woman in social interactions.

Women must speak out forcefully about the dangers of the obsession with thinness, says Kilbourne. "This is not a trivial issue; it cuts to the very heart of women's energy, power and self-esteem. This is a major public health problem, one that endangers the lives of young girls and women."

Women are dehumanized by beauty contests, body-building contests and pornography, as well as by advertisers and the fashion industry.
— Susan Kano

12. Effectiveness of treatment

If weight loss treatments are effective, why are so many people gaining weight instead of losing it?

The treatment of obesity is beyond the scope of this report, however, it is appropriate to consider briefly the odds for its success. Given the undeniable risks of intervention, the question needs to be asked of each treatment method if it will be successful enough to justify the risks it may entail.

In the past two decades Americans have made extraordinary efforts to lose weight. At any one time about 40 percent of women and 25 percent of men are trying to lose weight, spending $30 to $50 billion annually on weight loss products and services, according to the National Center for Health Statistics. Yet obesity has increased to a prevalence of 34 percent of adult Americans, up from 25 percent just a decade ago.[1]

If weight loss treatments are effective, why are so many people gaining weight instead of losing it?

The state of art in obesity treatment was summed up in 1958 by Albert Stunkard, MD, University of Pennsylvania, a pioneer in obesity research.

He said, "Most obese persons will not stay in treatment for obesity. Of those who stay in treatment, most will not lose weight, and of those who do lose weight, most will regain it."[1]

Since that time a great deal of evidence has been amassed that shows most people can lose considerable weight for a short time on various programs (or even a placebo).

The benefits for people with risk factors is marked.

Short-term benefits

The early benefits of weight loss for persons with risk factors related to obesity are well documented. Even a 10 to 15 percent weight loss or a four-week semi-starvation period can improve risk factors considerably.

A Harvard University study reported that with weight loss on a very low calorie diet, conditions were resolved for 34 percent of patients and improved for 23 percent of 154 diabetic patients. They were resolved for 39 percent and improved for 15 percent of 421 hypertensive patients. A weight loss of 5 percent of body weight was needed for improvement in cardiovascular conditions; 10 percent for improvement in diabetic and hypertensive conditions. A loss of at least 20 percent was needed to resolve conditions for half of diabetic and hypertensive patients.[2]

A Japanese study at Yokohama City University reported improved glucose intolerance in obese patients with diabetes and decreased fasting blood glucose, serum triglycerides and serum total cholesterol. The study investigated these risk factors for 57 severely obese patients with glucose intolerance during a four-week hospital stay.[3]

However, information on what happens next appears to be lacking. Four-weeks of improvement – or even a year – may be irrelevant in the life of a 40-year-old patient with a disease such as diabetes, particularly if adverse effects follow.

Some researchers say they believe reducing risk factors even for a

Grope in the dark

The public must understand that all current methods (for reducing weight), from thigh creams to stomach staples, are like gropes in the dark, and as such, are either totally ineffectual or are no more than counterforces to an incompletely understood regulatory disorder. There are no cures at this time.

The basic tenets of this industry are that there are commercially available programs that can safely lower body weight more easily than those of competitors and unlike their competitors, once the weight is lost, it will remain that way forever. On this basis, an endless set of new products, new diets, and drug interventions play legal tag with governmental regulatory agencies while reaping profit from a public desperate for answers.[S1]

– *Jules Hirsch*

short time is likely beneficial, but they provide no evidence.

The results of the almost inevitable weight regain are not at all clear. Is it beneficial over the longterm to reduce risk factors rapidly prior to an equally rapid rebound? Or is it harmful? What is the effect of weight cycling?

Much of this data is likely available and needs to be reported in the scientific literature. That it is not being reported may suggest that the longterm results are not favorable.

The Danish study

Long-term success of weight loss programs is rarely shown, particularly when measured by the Federal Trade Commission two-year definition.

In May 1991, FTC set the criteria that advertising of long-term effectiveness must be based on sound studies of least two years follow-up after the completion of the program. Later this was amended to include any maintenance within the program period. Thus the two years begins after the maintenance period, not before.

Very few of the many studies published each year in the scientific literature meet this criteria. Most "follow-ups" are one year or less, and many include part of the treatment program itself. Some actually begin the day the client signs up to lose weight.

It is widely reported in the popular press that 95 to 97 percent of weight loss efforts fail. There is little scientific evidence to refute this.

In a controlled study in Denmark, 57 patients were randomly assigned to very low calorie diet or horizontal gastroplasty surgery. They lost a great deal of weight in both programs.[4]

Their weight regain through five years is charted in *Figure 1* and *Figure 2 on page 102.*

By five years the success rate for VLCD was only 3 percent of patients. For surgery it was 16 percent. Success rate continued to decline, even for these subjects.

Success was defined modestly as keeping off 10 kg of their initial weight, or less than half of what they had lost. Success thus meant a modest reduction of from 264 pounds to 242 pounds for the average patient, or 8.3 percent of initial weight.

Few met this criteria of success after two years, and the numbers dropped each year, with no leveling off seen at any time.

Initial weight for the 57 patients was a median of 120 kg (264 lbs), 182 percent of ideal. Their maximum weight loss was reached at 9 months, with a median loss of 22 kg (48 lbs) for VLCD and 26 kg (57 lbs) for surgery.

The researchers could give no encouragement as to the effectiveness of either VLCD or gastric surgery. "Obviously, this outcome can satisfy neither professionals nor patients," they said.

Even though surgery gave somewhat better weight loss results than the diet, they concluded it was unjustified to continue to do the operation at their hospital because the complications and side effects were too numerous and serious.

San Diego study

Results of a long-awaited San Diego State University study on very

"Most obese persons will not stay in treatment for obesity. Of those who stay in treatment, most will not lose weight, and of those who do lose weight, most will regain it."
— Albert Stunkard

Figure 1

5 Year success rate in Denmark

	Years	% of patient success
VLCD	0-1	70
	1-2	38
	2-3	23
	3-4	8
	4-5	3
Gastroplasty	0-1	89
	1-2	66
	2-3	47
	3-4	24
	4-5	16

HEALTHY WEIGHT JOURNAL/O&H

Only 8 percent of the patients maintained as much as 41 percent of their weight loss for two years on VLCD.

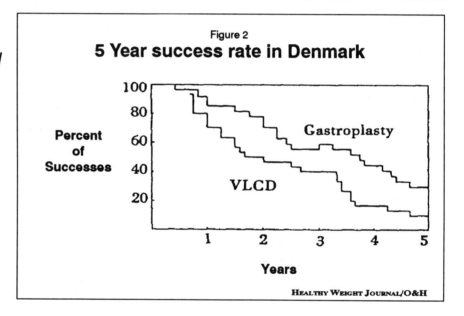

Figure 2

5 Year success rate in Denmark

HEALTHY WEIGHT JOURNAL/O&H

low calorie diets were equally disappointing.

In this study, 497 patients were randomly selected from a pool of 2,200 patients on the Optifast program. All were at least 25 pounds over desirable weight and had made at least two initial visits.

Only 8 percent of the patients maintained as much as 41 percent of their weight loss for two years. All groups, including these successful patients, were continuing to gain weight at two years, with no leveling off of weight gain. Over half of those in the study quit before completing the program (55 percent). The remaining 45 percent lost an average of 84 percent of their excess weight. (Men lost 63 pounds; women, 54 pounds.) But only one-fourth of the total number were able to keep off half their excess weight for nearly one year. Eight percent kept off less than half for two years.

However, the industry chose to report this study as a success. Information widely distributed through news channels and company clinics used key terms in confusing ways to indicate positive results.

For example, a news release reported, "The sample of patients who completed the 26-week treatment lost an average of 57 pounds, or 94 percent of their excess weight. When tracked after 18 months, 60 percent of patients sampled kept off an average of two-thirds of their loss. At 30 months, patients studied had kept off an average of 60 percent of their weight loss."

Patients who completed, patients sampled and *patients studied* actually refer to different, smaller and smaller groups. These are dwindling totals, although the reader is led to believe they are the same, or at least substantial groups. Further, the "follow-up" period reported as 30 months includes 26 weeks of treatment, so is actually only about 24 months.

One of the major researchers, Vincent Felitti, MD, said in the news release as saying, "Weight loss can now be easily, safely and routinely accomplished with a good probability of maintaining the loss. Five years ago this just wasn't the case. The frontier of dieting has moved from simply accomplishing a weight loss to maintaining the loss long term."

This industry report in 1988 was instrumental in convincing many physicians across the country to include very low calorie diets in their hospital programs.

Pennsylvania study

The benefits of rapid weight loss programs may be mostly wiped out in three years, say A. Stunkard, T. Wadden and J. Liebschutz, in a 1988 article in the *Journal of Consulting and Clinical Psychology.*[5]

In reporting a follow-up of their own much-quoted study, which showed excellent one-year results, they could only express disappointment.

The earlier study compared three programs: VLCD alone, behavior therapy alone, and the two combined. Weight loss was similar for all three. But at the end of the first year, a 12.9 kg (28 lb) weight loss was maintained for the combined group, compared with much less for the other two. Findings from this study were a major factor in the subsequent adding of behavioral components to most very low calorie diet programs.

In the three-year follow-up investigation, 45 of the 50 subjects were contacted. Forty percent had gone on other weight loss programs. The six who could be counted as "successful maintainers" had all been in repeated weight control efforts during the three years. Thus, failure to account for the intervening weight loss efforts would have led to overestimating long-term effectiveness, the researchers warn.

They also re-tested satisfaction scores, which had been very positive at the end of the first year. On a scale of 1 to 7, with 7 being most negative, scores dropped to between 5 and 6.4 on self-esteem, satisfaction with appearance, self-confidence, happiness, physical health, recreational activities, job performance, social activities, outlook for the future, sex life, and relationship with spouse/partner and family members. Depression scores, which had been much improved, were returned to original levels.

Moderate programs

Moderate programs are equally disappointing. (However, they may show marked improvement in diet, exercise and self-esteem factors over time, and are less likely to have adverse effects.)

The six successful maintainers had all been in repeated weight loss efforts during the intervening three years.

Obesity keeps scientists humble

Obesity continues to humble the scientific community by eluding effective understanding and intervention in many important respects.

The improvements that have been made in other areas of chronic diseases have occurred in spite of a continued high prevalence of obesity, not through an overall reduction in obesity-related risks.[53]
– *Shiriki Kumanyika*

In a report to the March 1992 NIH technology assessment conference on Methods for Voluntary Weight Loss and Control, John Foreyt, PhD, Baylor College of Medicine, said the average length of follow-up on behavioral treatment studies is one year, with about 66 percent of losses maintained for that period. Three to five year follow-ups show a gradual return to baseline.

Robert Jeffery, PhD, University of Minnesota, reported the results of community-based approaches at the NIH conference. He said the 10-year Minnesota Heart Health program was successful in delivering educational programs, counseling and referals, but could show no overall effect on weight. A comparison with other such interventions shows these results are typical, he said.

He also reported on a Minneapolis/St.Paul worksite program which enrolled 1,576 persons in weight loss. They lost an average of 2.2 kg over the six month program. However, there was no difference between treatment and control worksites in weight change.

New York City investigates

In 1991, following Congressional investigations of the weight loss industry, the New York City Department of Consumer Affairs did its own investigation of weight loss centers in New York. Among other findings reported elsewhere in this book, the DCA reported on effectiveness of weight loss programs.

Studies show that most dieters regain their weight, said the report, but sales representatives typically lead consumers to expect that their program will succeed on a long-term basis even if others have failed.

"The reality is we do not have effective treatment to offer, and we should be candid about this."
— Susan Wooley and David Garner

"In reality, no weight loss program can guarantee long-term success because programs do not monitor past clients on an ongoing basis. One may argue that keeping track of past clients isn't necessary; if the client faithfully follows the program, he or she will learn how to maintain their weight loss.

"There is a lack of demonstrated long-term benefits of very low calorie diets. Research shows that very low calorie diets fail because of the body's own physiological adaptation to a reduced caloric intake – not because the dieter returns to bad eating habits.

"A plan for long-term maintenance is nearly always stressed by the weight loss centers. What is not discussed, however, is that studies have shown that the majority of overweight people who lose weight regain it back within a few years.

"Weight loss centers often claim their success lies in helping the client change their behavior for life. They offer behavior modification classes to help the dieter learn, for example, what emotional cues trigger overeating.

"But the fact remains: there are no long-term studies to back up the claim that behavior modification works over the long haul, according to the American Medical Association's Council on Scientific Affairs. The findings of one five-year follow-up of 36 individuals who participated in a behavioral program for obesity showed a typical pattern of regaining all the weight lost during treatment.

"Diet programs will argue that their own studies show the weight loss is maintained. Most only gauge the dieter a year or less after the weight loss, according to Dr. (Wayne) Callaway. Medical authorities say a year is not long enough to determine if the program has really worked or not, and may only indicate one phase in a weight cycling pattern."

Integrity is needed

"It is difficult to find any scientific justification for the continued use of dietary treatments of obesity," according to David Garner, PhD, Michigan State University, and Susan Wooley, PhD, University of Cincinnati Medical Center, in a 1991 article in *Clinical Psychology Review.*[6]

"Regardless of the specific techniques used, most participants regain the weight lost. There is remarkable consistency in the pattern of regain across behavioral, dietary and very low calorie diet approaches to obesity. Most approaches lead to weight loss during active treatment, however, most participants ultimately regain to levels that approximate their pre-treatment weight."

Garner and Wooley say the inevitability of this result is often obscured by studies which claim success after a follow-up that is too short to show what really happens in later phases.

They charge that, contrary to scientific tradition which assumes there are no treatment effects until demonstrated, weight loss interventions are presumed effective until there is explicit evidence to the contrary.

"The reality is that we do not have effective treatment to offer, and we should be candid about this until there is reliable evidence to the contrary."

Some specialists are calling for more integrity and disclosure on the effectiveness of programs so consumers have a sound basis for making decisions. Much research receives funding from commercial weight loss companies, and this tends to add to the general confusion, frustration and complexity in the obesity field. It also contributes to the multiplicity of short-term studies in the literature, since short-term data shows the most favorable results for the program.

It is suggested that research on treatment could advance more quickly if researchers and treatment program directors would observe the FTC criteria and report at least two-year follow-up of their programs. It would also be helpful if editors of scientific journals would request two year follow-up data on the weight loss research they publish.

Studies which do provide long-term data offer much insight on why this is difficult and disheartening.

It soon becomes evident that, not only do most patients regain weight in two or three years, they launch many other dieting efforts. Their weight continues to fluctuate, up and down. Thus a follow-up can be very deceptive. In continuing weight cycles, some patients may be caught at a low weight, others at a peak, and still others midway between. The value in studying effectiveness of a specific program becomes lost in a long history of dieting and weight cycling. Nonetheless, it is clear that if the initial program were effective, there would be no need for others.

Weight loss methods vary from liquid diets to diet pills, meal supplements, stomach stapling, acupuncture, body wraps, rice diets, water diets, jaw wiring and hypnotism.

Why so many ways to lose weight? Quite plainly, the reason there are so many weight loss methods is because none of them really work. If even one of these lived up to its promise, there'd be no need for the

A doctor's weight loss education
by Allen King

For the past 20 years I have seen over 5,000 obese patients for weight reduction and weight related diseases. The results of my attempts to improve their disease state by weight loss were, at best, short-lived.

Initially, I thought obesity was caused by lack of knowledge. I gave patients an outline of the caloric content of foods. In a follow-up period of four weeks to four months, the average patient lost eight ounces. Half gained weight!

I next tried behavior modification and recruited a dietitian to provide a more individualized diet. In a three month follow up, the average patient lost only five pounds.

With the popular movement to liquid diets and their initial great success, I then tried a rigidly controlled program. Over 500 patients were placed on 500 to 1000 calorie diets with behavior modification. The average patient lost 50 pounds in six months. I felt we had finally succeeded. A three year follow up, however, uncovered an average 60 pound regain.

Certainly, I thought, what was needed was more control. Gastric surgeries were unacceptable due to the mortality and morbidity rate. Anorexic medications were of limited use. My two patients who elected jaw wiring lost weight initially, then regained. The Garren plastic balloon inflated in the stomach seemed the ideal solution. Weight loss did occur, but only in patients who developed ulcers and bowel obstructions.

I then became disillusioned and found myself avoiding discussing diet approaches with patients. Each method was followed by failure, and worse, guilt on the patient's part for "failing."

(King is currently using the nondiet approach and says this has allowed him to change from the diet, doctor-controlled model to self acceptance and removing masks for both patient and doctor.)[52]

others.

New guidelines at FTC

In the Congressional hearings, Chairman Wyden urged more aggressive action from federal regulatory agencies. "The diet indistry is now built on a foundation of false promises and false hopes," he said.[7]

In response, the Federal Trade Commission began an investigation of questionable marketing, advertising and service practices by diet companies. Six marketers of popular liquid diet programs and about a dozen other major diet companies were charged with making deceptive and unsubstantiated claims about their safety and effectiveness.

Such representations as the following (and many similar examples), were and are false and misleading, says the FTC:[8]

- "The focus is on long term sustained weight loss. In other words, what you lose stays lost." *(Optifast)*
- "You will not experience a rebound phenomenon (regain lost weight) after you attain your goal." *(Medifast)*
- "*Ultrafast* offers an effective maintenance program that enables you not only to lose the weight, but to keep it off!"

The FTC has established new guidelines for advertising weight loss programs and products, as follows:

1. **Claims that a certain weight loss is typical** must be based on a sample of all patients who have entered the program, or all persons who entered and completed the entire program or a portion thereof (where the claim only relates to such persons).
2. **Claims that weight loss is long term** must be based on the experience of patients followed for at least two years after they complete the program and maintenance program.
3. **Claims that weight loss is maintained permanently** must be based on a period of time generally recognized by experts as sufficient for such a claim, or for a period of time demonstrated by reliable survey evidence to permit such a prediction.
4. **Claims that patients have successfully maintained weight loss** need to include disclosures of average weight loss maintained by patients and how long they maintained it, as well as the statement, "For many dieters, weight loss is only temporary."

The March 1992 NIH Conference on Methods for Voluntary Weight Loss and Control issued a report which includes this warning on the ineffectiveness of weight loss programs: "For most weight loss methods, there are few scientific studies evaluating their effectiveness and safety. The available studies indicate that persons lose weight while participating in such programs but, after completing the program, tend to regain the weight over time. The lack of data on many commercial programs advertised for weight loss is especially disconcerting in view of the large number of Americans trying to lose weight and the over $30 billion spent yearly in America on weight loss efforts . . .

"Thus, the panel cautions that before individuals adopt any weight loss program, the scientific data on effectiveness and safety be examined. If no data exist, the panel recommends that the program not be used."

Claims that weight loss is longterm must be based on the experience of patients followed for at least two years.

— FTC

PART II

Challenges
for
Healthy
Change

13. To treat or not to treat

The question shocked medical sensibilities when Susan Wooley and O. Wayne Wooley asked in 1984, "Should obesity be treated at all?"

The question was posed in the scholarly text *Eating and Its Disorders.* For many years it was met primarily by silence, says Susan Wooley.[1]

Not only are diets and obesity treatment being challenged more frequently today, but the question has changed. Specialists are asking, "Are weight loss goals appropriate at all?"

Now the treatment issue has come full circle. Some health professionals suggest there is a need to treat dieting itself.

Immediate action is needed to "publicly identify dieting as a health risk equal in magnitude to other identifiable, treatable, and preventable risks such as cigarette smoking or unsafe sexual behavior," says Arnold Andersen, MD, an Iowa eating disorder specialist.[2]

"Our next frontier must be the . . . 'chronic dieting syndrome,' defined as a progressive pattern of frequent weight loss attempts followed by periods of discouragement and compulsive overeating," says Mike Bowers, PsyD, a Denver clinical psychologist. "The juggernaut of the dieting/overeating cycle and the accompanying distorted and polarized mindset destroys the person's sincere attempt at self-improvement and, in turn, destroys the hope of genuine success,"[3]

The powerful growth of the diet industry in the last two decades, its often questionable practices and false and misleading advertising, and the pressures to be thin has fueled concerns among many educators and health care providers that healthful solutions are not getting the attention they deserve.

"If treatment is not effective for healthy obese persons, why would it be effective for those at high risk?"
— David Garner

Dietitians at the 1991 American Dietetics Association annual meeting in Dallas were startled, but ready to listen when David Garner, PhD, a Michigan State University eating disorder specialist, told them, "It is difficult to find any scientific justification for the continued use of dietary treatments of obesity. The reality is that we do not have effective treatment to offer, and we should be candid about this until there is reliable evidence to the contrary."[4]

Two panel discussions on the subject *To Treat or Not to Treat* were presented at the 1992 conference and continuing education course of the North American Association for the Study of Obesity in Atlanta.

Since then the nondiet movement has grown. What began as a whisper was quickly picked up and embraced by the public: *"Diet's don't work!"* The diet industry, reeling from the blow, is fighting back.

Three viewpoints are expressed in the debate on this issue.

The first holds that the many current intervention methods, both radical and conservative, should continue. The rationale is that some methods may work better for some people and others for other people, and that more effective adaptations of these programs will likely be developed soon. This view is supported by the diet industry, industry-funded researchers in academia, and some health policy makers.

The second calls for a return to traditional, moderate weight management treatment, along with regulation of the weight loss industry. It advises against radical and rapid weight loss methods, which cause most injury.

The third view rejects all forms of weight loss treatment as not only ineffective, but harmful. It promotes health-oriented solutions with no emphasis on weight loss, which may or may not be an outcome.

Flawed logic

Garner takes the third view.

"The argument that health risk justifies treatment – in the absence of effective treatment – seems to me to be based upon flawed logic and is capricious. It doesn't make any sense that we should be trying to apply a treatment that's ineffective."

Garner points out that if a person is ill with cancer her physician does not treat her with laetrile, just because there is no cure. Yet unproven, risky treatments are used all too often with obesity problems.

Obesity treatment, until proven effective, should be held to the same standards as other treatments – on an experimental basis in controlled trials, says Garner. "The burden of proof should be on the people who are marketing the products. They should provide long-term follow-up data in support of the product before they make lots of money on it.

"I don't believe we should be offering mass merchandising of weight loss products based upon the flimsy evidence that exists for their efficacy. In fact there's strong evidence for them being ineffective."

Garner concedes his viewpoint has been described as radical, but protests that it is, in fact, very conservative. "It's just saying we should apply the same standards as are being applied to other treatments."

As for medical specialists who claim it is unethical not to treat obesity, Garner says, "I find that view preposterous. It flies in the face of everything else we do in medicine. We don't offer new forms of treatment until they're relatively safe and they're effective. Treatments are not just a sham."

Lifestyle change with weight loss

Other health professionals urge moderate weight loss treatment which helps people make lasting lifestyle changes, along with more emphasis on prevention.

For health care providers who would set weight goals for patients, such goals should be based on personal and family history, not on population-based mathematical models, cautions Karen Petersmarck, RD, Michigan Department of Public Health, editor of *Toward Safe Weight Loss: Recommendations for Adult Weight Loss Programs in Michigan*.[5]

Petersmarck says it is possible to mathematically predict a weight with the least risk of early mortality, based on population statistics, but it is not possible to define the optimal body weight for a given individual.

Health care providers should be certain that no harm is being caused by attempts to treat obesity, says F. Xavier Pi-Sunyer, MD, director of the Obesity Research Center, St. Luke's-Roosevelt Hospital in New York.

He cautions there is epidemiological evidence that weight loss and weight cycling may increase risk of mortality, even though it is well documented that obese individuals who lose weight improve their disease risk factors.

He urges professionals to be somewhat selective in accepting patients for weight loss treatment. The following overweight individuals, he suggests, could reasonably be treated:

■ Persons who are sick and whose illnesses are directly

"Our next frontier must be the . . . 'chronic dieting syndrome'
– Mike Bowers

alleviated by weight loss, such as non-insulin dependent diabetes.

- Persons with elevated risk factors for chronic disease such as hypercholesterolemia and hypertension.
- Persons with family histories of chronic disease and high waist-to-hip ratios.[6]

At what point should weight loss intervention begin?

This is a viable medical question in dealing with severe risk factors related to obesity.

Some would define the point at which a radical solution is reasonable, given the risk factors, at 130 to 140 percent of optimal weight. Others, more conservatively, say an excess of 100 pounds, and still others, when medical risk factors are present.

However, leaders in the nondiet movement disagree.

If treatment is not effective for moderately obese persons in good health, they ask, why would it be effective for those who are severely obese or at high risk? And when the treatment offered is not only ineffective, but appears to have serious health risks, how can professionals ethically subject to it persons who are already at risk?

"The logic fails. You have a very temporary relief, followed by a sharp increase in health risk factors. There is potential for both health risk and mortality risk when you have big weight fluctuations," Garner points out.

Nondiet movement gains strength

From the turmoil of widespread frustration with diets that don't work, pressures to be thin, and the crises in eating disorders that grips America, a new movement is rising. It is a paradigm shift, vigorously opposed to dieting.[7]

The nondiet approach to weight problems focuses on wellness solutions, not weight loss.

Most treatment programs that use this approach focus on three factors: feeling good about oneself, eating well in a natural, relaxed way, and being comfortably active.

It is not possible to define the optimal body weight for a given individual.
— Karen Petersmarck

This new movement advocates no dieting, no food restraint, and instead promotes helping people learn to eat in natural ways. It teaches an awareness of hunger and how to respond to internal signals, not eating prescribed foods at specified times.

This approach focuses on self-discovery, not will power; on self-esteem, diversity and accepting people as they are, not judging; with getting on with one's life, not waiting to be thin.

The nondiet approach challenges old rules for weight loss, as well as the current direction taken by fitness and wellness programs. A few new programs have been developed.

Linda Omichinski, RD, a Canadian dietitian and leader in the nondiet movement, compares the nondiet and the traditional diet approaches. The differences are, she says, self-discovery versus compliance, empowerment versus control, and feelings of well-being versus failure in maintaining weight loss. In the nondiet model the individual is in control, in the diet model, the health professional.

"It means finding the strength to accept yourself just as you are and get on with life." Omichinski is the author of *You Count, Calories Don't,* and the *Hugs Facilitator Kit,* a nondiet program for health care leaders.[8]

Ellyn Satter, MS, RD, a Wisconsin dietitian, psychotherapist and eating specialist, defines *normal eating* as "being able to eat when you are hungry and continue eating until you are satisfied," and "eating primarily in response to internal cues of hunger, appetite and satiety."

Author of bestselling books for parents *How to Get Your Kid to Eat – But Not Too Much*, and *Child of Mine*, Satter emphasizes the need for people of all ages to learn positive and natural ways of managing their eating. Her workshops on "Treating the Dieting Casualty," are designed to help people replace distorted eating with normal eating.[9]

The Overcoming Overeating workshops led by therapists Jane Hirschmann and Carol Munter, authors of *When Women Stop Hating Their Bodies* and *Overcoming Overeating*, are also aimed at breaking the dieting cycle. Women must stop torturing themselves over food, say Hirschmann and Munter. "The time has come for us to stop the dieting that has become a life-long, life-draining preoccupation. Dieting has turned millions of us into food junkies, driven, compulsive eaters who grow fatter every year. The time has come for us to enjoy our bodies in all their diversity. The time has come for us to reclaim our appetites, our bodies, and our lives."[10]

A fresh approach to exercise is also part of the new nondiet paradigm. Too often exercise has been viewed as a new religion that glorifies muscles and sweat, says Gail Johnston, a California health and fitness

"Normal eating is being able to eat when you are hungry and continue eating until you are satisfied."
— Ellyn Satter

Diet vs. nondiet thinking on key issues

ISSUE	DIET THINKING	NONDIET THINKING
Goal	weight loss	confidence in ability to make choices for better health
Progress	any weight loss	gradual life-style changes
Self Acceptance	only after weight loss is achieved	starts the natural self-nurturing cycle
Success	goal weight	energetic daily living, increased self-esteem
Exercise	no pain, no gain; should, shouldn't	get hooked on increasing activity; fun and energy
Food	food is the enemy; deprivation; willpower	food is the friend; celebrate; enjoy; taste; savor
Language	Should I have it?; Do I need it?	Do I want it?
Thinking	all or nothing – "I can have it all or nothing at all"	"I can have it if I really want it."
Attitude	perfectionist; must be a certain way	flexible; goes with the flow
Choice	diet in control; no choice	person in charge; decides what and when to eat
Hunger	out of touch with physical hunger – may eat in response to psychological hunger, ie. when under stress	in tune with body's internal cues of physical hunger; listens to body; does not turn to food when dealing with problems such as stress

Reprinted with permission from You Count, Calories Don't, and HUGS Facilitator Kit, by Linda Omichinski. Copyright 1992, 1993, 1994.

HUGS™/HEALTHY WEIGHT JOURNAL/O& H

consultant.

A better approach is more relaxed, she suggests. It focuses on exercise as a pleasurable experience, an activity in which everyone can succeed and work into their daily life. It is not necessary to count heart rate or work up to training levels, Johnston says. Nor is it necessary to lose weight to achieve the benefits of exercise.[11]

Enthusiasm for the new programs is growing fast among nutrition and eating disorder professional groups.

The Society for Nutrition Education affirmed its support for this approach in a 1994 letter to former Attorney General C. Everett Koop in declining his request to join the "Shape Up America" campaign.

"We support a new weight paradigm that opposes fat phobia, deals honestly with the difficulties of long term maintenance of weight loss, accepts the goal of health promotion and quality of life rather than slenderness, and recognizes the rights of heavy persons to make decisions about their own goals and behaviors," said the letter from SNE's Advisory Committee on Partnerships.

In Quebec a professional dietitians' group, Corporation Proffesionnelle des Dietetistes du Quebec, issued a statement in 1992 that emphasized the need for healthy standards, "We must intervene without making the situation worse. To this end, the CPDQ wishes to see, instead of a group of diet victims, a population of varied size, good physical and mental health."[12]

A new organization for clinicians who work with large patients using the nondiet approach is AHELP (Association for the Health Enrichment of Large Persons), formed in 1991. It promotes health-based treatment and research into ways large people can be helped without

> *"It means finding the strength to accept yourself just as you are and get on with life."*
> — Linda Omichinski

Obesity treatment without harm

Statement by Corporation professionnelle des dietetistes du Quebec

To help individuals reach and/or maintain a healthy weight, practice enjoyable physical activities, and develop healthy eating habits while respecting their traditions, tastes and lifestyles, CPDQ recommends:

1. Use healthy body weight standards to evaluate body weight and the waist-hip ratio to assess health risks.
2. Take into account overall lifestyle when a person feels uneasy about self: weight may not be the cause. Other changes more relevant may be stopping smoking, increasing physical activity, relaxation or making better food choices.
3. Don't be too influenced by social pressures and body norms. Do not be afraid to maintain your own healthy body weight or to keep a few curves if it suits you better.
4. Where an objective evaluation indicates a significant excess weight in the abdominal region:
   a. Analyze reasons for deciding to lose weight. It is better to wait and succeed than to start something bound to fail. Losing weight is not a game.
   b. Make simple and reasonable changes. Be patient. When motivated, it is possible to lose weight by a slight decrease in food intake, better food choices

and participating in the physical activities of your preference.
   c. Seek a competent professional if you encounter difficulties with the steps described above.

CPDQ warns against:

- seeking a body weight which is too low for good health;
- products and diets not tailored to the individual;
- risks to physical and mental health which can be greater than those related to the excess weight.

Dietitians would like to help people who suffer from obesity to lose weight and maintain their healthy weight so as to assure them a potential for the best health possible. However, reality is very different and without guaranteed success.

We must intervene without making the situation worse. To this end, the CPDQ wishes to see, instead of a group of diet victims, a population of varied size, good physical and mental health.

Excerpted from the Timely Statement on The Treatment of Obesity, Apr 28, 1992.[13]

---

weight loss. Goals are to develop a new theoretical foundation with "more creative options to help move obese persons into the direction of self-acceptance and health restoration rather than merely counting pounds lost as an indicator of self-esteem and treatment success."

The group aims to alter the thinking of health care providers who stigmatize large people into dieting, forcing their patients into unhealthy practices and promoting self-hate.

Joe McVoy, PhD, a founder of AHELP and an eating disorder specialist in Virginia, says, "We feel that the societal prejudice against fat people, and weight loss through dieting have most harmful effects. Consequently, we actively oppose fatism within both our profession and our society, and oppose food restriction for weight loss."

Therapists and doctors often do damage to the emotional and physical health of large patients through their treatment of them, he warns. "Health professionals have the greatest potential for harm, but they also have the greatest potential for change."[14]

Shifting national policy

Canada is in the forefront of the effort to shift focus from weight loss to health-oriented solutions, thanks to the research and dedication of eating disorder specialists such as Janet Polivy, PhD, and Peter Herman, PhD, at the University of Toronto. Canada has initiated a policy advocating the acceptance of a broad range of healthy weights and health related programs for people of every weight.

In 1988, Health and Welfare Canada issued challenges to both consumers and professionals to make healthy changes in five major areas (attitude, lifestyle, treatment, environment, knowledge) to deal more effectively with weightism and the problems of obesity.[15]

Canadian health care workers were issued a clear warning: *If you cannot help, at least do no harm.*

A nation-wide Canadian health program *Vitality* combines the three components of the nondiet, health-based paradigm – feeling good about oneself, eating well, and being active. The *Vitality* program de-emphasizes weight, and fosters self-empowerment within the social environment. Its preventive efforts are intended to initially focus on young adults, age 25 to 44. This is the age group considered to have the most influence for helping others change, as well as being at high risk for developing heart disease, cancer and diabetes.

Continuing its own somewhat heavy-handed policy, the U.S. Public Health Service was then, in the late 1980s, increasing pressures to be thin. Health objectives for the nation included the directive that 50 percent of overweight Americans should be on weight loss regimens by 1990.[16]

However, U.S. health objectives for the year 2000 represent an attitude change at policy-making levels. The Healthy People 2000 objectives acknowledge the complexity of obesity, while calling for a reduction in the prevalence of overweight to 20 percent for adults and 15 percent for adolescents.

"We must intervene without making the situation worse . . . instead of a group of diet victims, a population of varied size, good physical and mental health."
– Quebec dietitians

14. Diet industry regulation

The weight loss industry is a $30 to $50 billion health-related business which profoundly affects the health of many citizens. Each year it is associated with many deaths and severe injuries. Yet it is not regulated, or held accountable in any way for its outcomes.

Public impatience with the weight loss industry found a national focus when a congressional subcommittee held hearings in 1990. Chaired by Rep. Ron Wyden, (D-Ore.), the hearings found many abuses and revealed that federal agencies were lax in enforcing food, drug, and advertising laws related to weight loss. "Sleeping watchdogs," Wyden called them.

As a result, the Food and Drug Administration did take action to ban 111 diet pill ingredients for nonprescription sales in 1992, an action delayed for nearly 20 years. The Federal Trade Commission, which is responsible for truth in advertising, initiated aggressive action over the next few years against nearly all the companies engaged in marketing diet products and services, both large and small. Eventually most were charged with false and misleading advertising, and signed consent agreements. This action continues and as a result, most advertising claims have become less blatant.

New York City conducted an extensive investigation of weight loss centers in the city and, in 1993 set up requirements for the posting of warnings and consumer rights.

This was followed by similar action that introduced legislation into the New York State Assembly in 1993-1994, under the chairmanship of Sen. William Bianchi, Task Force on Food, Farm and Nutrition Policy.

"There are no recognized standards of care, no establiished criteria for health monitoring or medical supervision, and no accountability in reporting injury or death.
— Michigan Task Force

Recommendations for consumer protection

Consumers need more protection, C. Wayne Callaway, MD, associate clinical professor of medicine at George Washington University, testifying for the American Board of Nutrition, said at the 1990 congressional hearing. Commercial weight loss programs are "skillfully and deliberately exploiting a situation where cultural norms are dramatically out of 'sync' with biological reality," he said.

Callaway made the following recommendations for regulating the weight loss industry and protecting consumers:[1]

1. Public information. Establish an effective mechanism for tracking the incidence and severity of complications of unsupervised and poorly supervised weight loss programs. Create a clearinghouse for collecting reports of adverse effects and for making this information available to the public, as well as more information on the hazards and lack of demonstrated long-term benefits of very low calorie diets.

2. Accountability. Weight loss programs should be responsible for their outcomes. Documented complications, such as the high incidence of gallstone formation during low calorie diets, cannot be simply dismissed as due to the dieter's obesity. Similarly, if most dieters regain the weight they have lost on commercially available programs, the dieter can no longer be blamed.

3. Trained medical supervision. Severely restricted diets should be undertaken only by people for whom there is a clear and urgent medical reason. In all cases such treatment should be supervised by physicians who have both the training and knowledge to recognize and treat effectively the complications of semi-starvation.

4. Standardized reporting. All weight loss programs should be required to track their outcome data and to analyze and publish such data in an open, verifiable way. Standardized data collection and reporting would allow the real risks and costs, versus long-term benefits of different weight reduction approaches to be assessed.

5. Promote healthy weight. Science and the media need to advance the idea of individualized healthy weights, rather than continuing to promote the unhealthy cultural distortion that has led to our current epidemic of dieting. People are of different sizes and shapes, just as they have different skin colors and ethnic backgrounds. Biological variability is not regarded as a disease, but as one of the strengths of the human species.

The industry includes "a new mix of questionable products, untrained providers and deceptive advertising, exposing our citizens to unexpected health risks," Wyden charged.

Somewhat earlier, the Michigan Health Council Task Force published a report *Toward Safe Weight Loss*, in response to concern over seven documented Michigan deaths associated with dieting programs. Endorsed by 45 health care Michigan organizations, the report said obesity should be regarded as a medical problem requiring appropriate and professional health care, and recommended all weight loss programs be considered health programs and meet required standards.[2] It noted that the weight loss industry is not regulated by any state or federal agency, and there are no recognized standards of care, no established criteria for health monitoring or medical supervision, and no accountability in reporting injury or death.

The Task Force also recommended setting treatment standards to include client screening and full written disclosure of all phases of the program including long-term results, and requiring that claims be backed by sound research.

New York City takes the first step

In the first-ever such action in the U.S., New York City in 1993 took a strong step in regulating the weight loss industry.

The new rules require disclosure of the consumers' right to know the details of a program, its health risks, costs, qualifications of staff, and the dangers of rapid weight loss.[3]

The action was prompted by a New York City Department of Consumer Affairs investigation which revealed numerous "dangerous and deceptions" in weight loss centers and programs. It found that often customers were not given accurate information about programs and costs. Nor were they warned of the dangers associated with major weight loss, "although weight loss centers know of the health risks."

Weight loss centers are big business in New York with at least nine major weight loss services and scores of branches in the metropolitan region, says the report. Yet "they are not regulated by any state or local authority."

The Consumer Affairs department researched three segments of

Providers of appropriate programs can only be strengthened by reasonable regulation and accountability, instead of – as now – being continually undermined by the irresponsibile behavior of others.

New York City regulates weight loss centers

Disclosure to consumers

The Department of Consumer Affairs has monitored the unregulated rapid weight loss industry and found that it fails to adequately warn potential clients of health risks and adverse side effects associated with rapid weight loss programs. Awareness of such health risks and adverse side effects can enable potential clients to better select programs based on an informed choice.

The potential damage caused by rapid weight loss programs is a serious health issue which must be confronted and dealt with immediately.

Rapid weight loss centers usually fail to disclose to potential clients that rapid weight loss, as a means of treatment of obesity, can result in heart injury, gallbladder injury, and several other serious conditions. They typically do not warn consumers in advance or openly discuss potential dangers and side effects with consumers, and the consumer remains unaware of the potential side effects which may be experienced only after the consumer starts the program.

The purpose of the proposed rule is to alert consumers to the dangers involved in rapid weight loss.

First, the proposed rule will require weight loss centers to post a public notice warning consumers that there may be potential side effects and health risks associated with rapid weight loss. The notice would also inform consumers that only permanent lifestyle changes such as healthful food choices and increasing physical activity promote permanent weight loss.

Second, the weight loss provider must distribute a palm-sized card which the consumer may take home so that he/she may further consider the risks and benefits of the weight loss program.

Third, the proposed rule will require weight loss providers to disclose additional charges that a consumer may incur for the purchase of products and the cost of laboratory tests in seeking to achieve his or her weight loss goals.

Fourth, the proposed rule will require weight loss providers to tell consumers what the actual or estimated duration of their recommended program will be.

Fair trade practices

A. A "weight loss provider" is defined as any person or business entity who or which is primarily engaged in the business of offering services to consumers to assist them in losing weight.

B. It is a deceptive trade practice for a weight loss provider to quote to a consumer a fixed or estimated cost for a weight loss program that is being recommended for the particular consumer without separately stating any additional charges the consumer may have to pay to purchase products, services, supplements or laboratory tests which are part of such program.

C. It is a deceptive trade practice for a weight loss provider to recommend a weight loss program to a particular consumer without also disclosing the actual or estimated duration of the program.

D. It is a deceptive trade practice for a weight loss provider to make any oral or written statement, visual description or other representation of any kind, including in any advertisement, which statement, description or representation has the capacity, tendency or effect of leading consumers to believe that the use of a product or treatment, or participation in a program, will result in weight loss unless the weight loss provider conspicuously posts the following statement in each of its weight loss establishments: *(See poster on page 53.)*

E. The above statement *[see poster]* must be posted in a notice to the public at every temporary or permanent location of the weight loss provider. The notice must be conspicuously posted in every room in which a presentation is made, or in which a product or treatment is offered for sale, by the weight loss provider. The notice must be printed in letters at least in 36 point bold face type on a sign at least 22 inches by 34 inches in size. The sign shall be entitled "Weight Loss Consumer Bill of Rights" which shall be printed in letters of 60 point bold face type.

F. All the educational and professional experience of the weight loss provider's staff must be made available upon the request of any person.

G. Every weight loss provider shall produce and distribute to all consumers who inquire about its weight loss program a palm-sized card entitled "Weight Loss Consumer Bill of Rights," which shall contain the same information contained in the poster described in subdivision **D.** above.

H. Every weight loss provider shall post the sign described in subdivision **D.** which shall be provided by the Department of Consumer Affairs, and shall reproduce and distribute the palm-sized card described in subdivision **G.**, in every location in which its program or product is promoted, presented or sold, and the weight loss provider must cause the posting of such sign and the distribution of such card by every agent, representative, franchisee and independent contractor at every location in which such agent, representative, franchisee or independent contractor promotes, presents or sells the weight loss provider's program or product.[4]

Note: An amendment later decreased the size of the sign to 22 1/2 by 17 1/2 inches, required it to include the Department of Consumer Affairs name, address and telephone, and permitted the weight loss providers to include their names, addresses and telephone numbers, in print no larger than the letters used in the main text of the sign or card.

For more information contact: New York City Department of Consumer Affairs, Mark Green, Commissioner, 80 Lafayette St., New York, NY 10013 (212-788-4636).

the commercial weight loss industry:

- Rapid weight loss programs in which the person fasts on liquid formula, "supposedly supervised by physicians and hospitals."
- Commercial weight loss centers that restrict the diet through regimented meal plans.
- Commercial meal-replacement powders.

Posing as potential clients, the DCA staff called or visited 14 weight loss centers. They found:

- Nine out of ten surveyed centers did not give advance warning or openly discuss the potential safety risks involved in their specific program or of rapid weight loss in general, even when asked directly about possible health problems.
- Some weight loss centers attempted to sell their weight loss services to people who did not need them – including the underweight. (One underweight woman was told she could lose five pounds, which would have put her statistically at risk for certain medical problems.)
- Some weight loss centers are engaged "more in quackery than medicine. At one clinic we were told that gorging on certain foods could speed up metabolism."
- Some centers subject prospective customers to high pressure sales tactics that "verge on harassment."

Some weight loss centers are engaged "more in quackery than medicine."
– NYC Consumer Affairs

The report which came out of this investigation, *A Weighty Issue: Dangers and Deceptions of the Weight Loss Industry,* cites numerous dangers and potential side effects, of rapid weight loss in particular, and questions the qualifications of many staff.

While the range of services that diet programs offer varies, says the report, so do the experience and qualifications of the people who run them. "In the liquid diet segment in those medically-supervised programs, the qualifications of the doctors may run the gamut of experience:

(A POSTER)

Weight Loss Consumer Bill of Rights

1. WARNING: Rapid weight loss may cause serious health problems. (Rapid weight loss is weight loss of more than 1 1/2 pounds to 2 pounds per week or weight loss of more than 1 percent of body weight per week after the second week of participation in a weight loss program.)

2. Only permanent lifestyle changes – such as making healthful food choices and increasing physical activity – promote long-term weight loss.

3. Consult your personal physician before starting any weight loss program.

4. Qualifications of this provider's staff are available on request.

5. You have a right to:
   i. ask questions about the potential health risks of this program, its nutritional content, and its psychological-support and educational components;
   ii. know the price of treatment, including the price of any extra products, services, supplements and laboratory tests: and
   iii. know the program duration that is being recommended for you.

New York City requires that a poster with this information (22 1/2 x 17 1/2 in.) be displayed by weight loss providers.[5]

HWJ/OBESITY & HEALTH 1993

New York State proposal

Registration of advertisers of weight loss services:

1. Any person, firm, or corporation offering weight loss services in this state by means of advertising such services to the public shall annually register with the state board of dietetics and nutrition and submit the following information to the department:

  a. training and qualifications of personnel providing counseling and other weight loss services,

  b. ingredient and nutrition information for any food, formula or drug product sold or provided as part of a weight loss program,

  c. an explanation of how claims for weight loss will be achieved by the services advertised, and

  d. if the service has been offered for one year of more:

   i. a record of the number of clients in the previous year who have successfully achieved weight loss according to the program's goals,

   ii. the total number of clients served during the previous year, and

   iii. the number of clients who have reported medical problems related to the weight loss services.

2. Every person, firm or corporation registering pursuant to this section, shall be charged a fee of twenty-five dollars upon registering.

3. The state board of dietetics and nutrition shall compile this information and make it available to the public in a report to be issued by May 1 of each year. Information shall be furnished to any person upon request.

4. The state board of dietetics and nutrition may periodically review client records of persons, firms, or corporations advertising weight loss services to verify the accuracy of the information submitted.

NY State Assembly, Bill 6703, Sec 8003-a.[81]

New York State. Contact: Bob Stern, Director Task Force on Food, Farm & Nutrition Policy, NY State Assembly, State Capitol, Albany, NY 12248 (518-455-5203.)

some weight loss physicians are seasoned physicians with advanced training in nutrition while others may have only received rudimentary nutrition courses at a medical school. Some programs offer nutritional counseling by registered dietitians; others use nonprofessionals such as ex-clients."

Generally, the customers are led to believe they are receiving a health-care service, said the report, but in the "commercially-driven atmosphere, too often the center's goal becomes sales, not health."

Even diet programs affiliated with physicians and hospitals may be more interested in generating profit than providing quality treatment, the investigators found.

False claims

The report recognized the vulnerability and desperation of the customer. "The daily barrage of commercials and television shows emphasizing thinness as an ideal reinforces the message that overweight people don't fit into society. Their vulnerability makes them easy targets for diet services promising quick results and an end to their low self esteem," said the New York City report.

However, "There is a lack of demonstrated long-term benefits . . . Sales representatives typically lead consumers to expect that their program will succeed on a long-term basis even if others have failed. But in reality, no weight loss program can guarantee long-term success because programs do not monitor past clients on an ongoing basis. One may argue that keeping track of past clients isn't necessary; if the client faithfully follows the program, he or she will learn how to maintain their weight loss. But research shows that very low calorie diets fail because of the body's own physiological adaptation to a reduced caloric intake – not because the dieter returns to bad eating habits.

"A plan for long-term maintenance is nearly always stressed by the weight loss centers. What is not discussed, however, is that studies have shown that the majority of overweight people who lose weight regain it back within a few years."

New York City Consumer Affairs Commissioner Mark Green said the diet industry has seen a huge growth in the past decade along with a "rising tide of questionable practices."

Green called for accountability. "There are currently no federal regulations to oversee the maze of diet programs out on the market, nor are there any minimum standards for operating such programs. Consumers often mistakenly believe that diet clinics are licensed, but in fact, they are not regulated by an state or local authority."

The new rules require posting warnings and disclosure information in all weight loss centers in New York City.

New York State seeks new laws

Two bills seeking to regulate the weight loss industry were introduced into the 1993-1994 State of New York Assembly. The first bill is similar to the New York City rules on posting consumer warnings and disclosure of qualifications of providers. The second bill requires registration of advertisers of weight loss services. The two bills are still being debated in 1995, according to Bob Stern, Director of the Task Force on Food, Farm and Nutrition Policy, Committee on Consumer Affairs and

Protection.[6]

While they have not passed the assembly, these bills may be useful as model legislation elsewhere. The sponsors made the following justifications for the bills.

"Millions of New Yorkers have tried or are trying to lose weight for medical and cosmetic reasons. Unfortunately the results of medical research about the safety and effectiveness of diet programs are often vague and even contradictory. There is very little regulation of this industry. This makes it difficult for consumers to decide what programs and products to use.

"Although commercial diets have received little attention in the past, recent reports about high rates of gallbladder disease in clients of certain programs has heightened concern about medical complications. Studies of dieters who continually lose and then regain weight, the so called 'yo-yo' effect, show increased risk of heart disease and other problems. Many programs and products are offered or sold by celebrities, health 'experts,' store clerks and others who have no background or training in nutrition and health. Those offering the services sometimes advertise quick solutions that may be risky."[7]

In testimony at the New York State Assembly public hearing in late 1993, Bianchi said consumers need to be warned of the potential risks involved in weight loss.

"Weight loss businesses should clearly explain to the consumers how their program or product is supposed to work and the qualifications for the staff. If a company is going to make a claim about the success of their program or product, they should be able to back it up with statistics or research. Consumers want to know if a program or product is going to work. Even the best diet programs that recommend safe diets don't work very well. Unfortunately, some weight loss companies lead people to believe that they aren't trying hard enough or they haven't found the right diet. Advertisements for diet programs and products are filled with success stories, but we don't see the dropout rates or the long term weight loss of the average client," Bianchi said.

Unscrupulous doctors are part of the problem, charged Louis J. Aronne, MD, physician and assistant professor of medicine at Cornell U Medical College, director of a weight control center at the New York Hospital. He testified that the reason insurance companies often refuse payment for obesity treatment is partly because the results are so poor, and partly because of the "relatively high level of outright fraud in physician-supervised obesity treatment." He said it was clear the medical profession does not police itself very well.

He gave an example of a case in which a physician claimed his weight loss program was covered by insurance. Initially, patients were given tests costing $2,000 billed to the insurance company, and then received a two-page preprinted diet. "All these people were completely healthy and had no need to have any of the tests," said Aronne.

In another case, a female undercover agent weighing 120 pounds went to a physician advertising weight loss. "He said very little to her, gave her a prescription for diet pills, for which he then gave her a fraudulent bill," he said. "These guys know nothing about anything. All they know is that you can sell diet pills by advertising that you have a weight control program."

For some reason, said Aronne, physicians are susceptible to this.

"The diet industry has seen a huge growth in the past decade along with a rising tide of questionable practices."
— Mark Green

"Weight loss programs should be responsible for their outcomes . . . if dieters regain, (they) can no longer be blamed."
– C. Wayne Callaway

But he strongly recommended the services of dietitians in weight management. "To the best of my knowledge, the most responsible treaters of obesity as a group have been the dietitians. This does not happen with dietitians, because that's sort of ingrained in them that the right thing to do is to get (patients) to exercise and put them on a food based diet, and if that were the first line of treatment in all weight control programs, you would have much less of the nonsense that we see."

Aronne recommended that "every person, including physicians and other health care professionals who claim to treat obesity, be subjected to the same requirements, including registration."

Advertising is another problem, Aronne testified at the hearing. "A huge weight control industry has developed in which the marketers of products, including physicians, create the illusion that they have the secret to weight control success by showing one person, usually a celebrity, who has succeeded, however briefly. This type of advertising verges on exploitation, because those with the disease of obesity are desperate to get rid of it and want to believe that someone has the answer, the more magical the better."

The consumer's right to know

Clearly an idea whose time has come, regulation of the weight loss industry is moving closer to reality. Regulation of weight loss services and products is long overdue. Providers of appropriate weight management programs can look forward to having reasonable regulation and accountability guidelines. They can only be strengthened by such regulation, instead of – as now – being continually undermined by the irresponsible behavior of others.

Action has been taken toward regulation in the following five critical areas.

1. **Disclosure to consumers**
   - New York City regulations require weight loss providers to
   Post warnings on risks and the need for long-term lifestyle changes.
   Post information on the right to know full details on program, risks and staff qualifications before purchase
   - A New York State bill proposes to
   Require advertisers of weight loss services and products to post, provide to consumers, and include in all advertising certain warnings.
   Make available upon request the required registration information.
2. **Advertising**
   - The Federal Trade Commission's charges of false and misleading advertising against six liquid diet companies suggest that FTC intends to require that:
   Claims of safety and effectiveness be verified by scientific data.
   Claims of long-term weight loss be based on results at least two years after the program ends, including maintenance.
   Testimonials and weight loss claims represent the typical experience of those who enter the program.
3. **State registration**
   - A New York State bill calls for registration of all those who advertise weight loss services, including full program information and staff qualifications (action pending).

4. **Accreditation**
- An industry plan, spearheaded by Arthur Frank, MD, Obesity Management Program, George Washington University, would set standards for voluntary accreditation of weight loss programs through a self-sustaining, non-government board similar to the hospital system. It would likely develop levels of treatment, with specific care, services and provider training set at each level.

5. **Accountability**
- The New York State proposal would require advertisers, after one year of operation, to provide figures on the number of clients served, the number who have achieved weight loss goals, and the number who have reported medical problems related to the weight loss services.[6]

"The most responsible treaters of obesity as a group have been the dietitians."
— Louis Aronne

15. Challenges for wellness and wholeness

*We can no longer permit
these critical decisions
to be made
by people who refuse
to consider the effect
their decisions
may have on women
and on persons
of all sizes, or
who serve
the weight loss industry.*

A major health challenge of the decade is how to reconcile the tough issues of weight. How can we prevent eating disorders without increasing the rates of obesity? How can we prevent obesity without increasing disordered eating, thinness obsession and size discrimination?

The challenges of weight involve complex and difficult issues reaching all the way across the weight spectrum. We are in the midst of a national weight crisis, and at high risk for further detrimental effects.

Problems that have been ignored too long are becoming more acute. They include the following critical issues:

■ Eating disorder risks

An estimated 10 percent of students in the United States have eating disorders, most of them female. Studies find a death rate as high as 18 percent from anorexia nervosa and bulimia nervosa. Disordered eating may be the norm for pre-adolescent girls; a California study finds 80 percent of 10- to 11-year-olds affected.

■ Obesity risks

Obesity has increased to a prevalence of 34 percent of U.S. adults and 21 percent of adolescents, and has shown a rapid rise among children. It is associated with five of the ten leading causes of death in the U.S., as well as many other diseases and conditions. Related health problems are especially acute among minority and low income populations. Costs reach $100 billion annually.

■ Risks of treatment

As documented in this report, dieting and weight loss attempts can result in numerous adverse effects. Among these are sudden death, gallstones, cardiac disorders, elevated cholesterol, anemia, fatigue, hair loss, nausea, cold intolerance, changes in liver function and amenorrhea. Psychological risks include depression, apathy, irritability, moodiness, anxiety, low self-esteem, rigidity and inability to concentrate. There is little evidence of longterm effectiveness for any of the many weight loss methods in use.

■ Obsession with thinness

Currently there is intense pressure to be extremely thin. Miss America contestants and Playboy centerfold girls have become progressively thinner over 30 years; they are now at 13 to 18 percent below expected weight, a criteria for anorexia nervosa. Even elite female Olympic gymnasts average only about 90 pounds. This has led to intense dieting efforts. About 40 percent of women and 25 percent of men are trying to lose weight at any one time, many using potentially dangerous methods such as diet pills, laxatives, diuretics, vomiting, fasting or semi-starvation.

■ Size discrimination

Prejudice can be severe against large persons in employment, education, health care and social relationships. Discrimination limits the lives of many large persons and may delay medical care.

■ Industry unregulated

Weight loss is a $30 to $50 billion health-related industry which is not regulated or held accountable for its outcomes. Injuries and death are not reported. Exploitation, false advertising, exorbitant profits, and outright fraud are widespread.

■ Women's issues ignored

Women's issues are critical to weight problems. They include eating disorders, dieting, sexual abuse, obsession with thinness, size prejudice, and the sometimes-large weight gains of adolescence, pregnancy and menopause. Yet these factors are being ignored.

■ Research fragmented

A major obstacle to meeting the crisis effectively is the fragmentation of weight studies into many academic disciplines and national disease centers, which generally place their emphasis on other areas. None deal with weight issues in a unified, comprehensive way. Some of these are nutrition, medicine, psychology, public health and physical education and research centers devoted to cardiovascular disease and diabetes.

All these factors are in the mix when we view the complex area of weight and what it means in our culture. The risks of both eating disorders and obesity are more urgent than ever – "epidemics" have been declared. Most professionals deal with only a few elements, sometimes working at cross-purposes with one another, while the crisis grows. This nation has not dealt well with weight issues in the past. Health policy tends to react to events in specific areas, rather than addressing the real issues in a comprehensive way. Attempts to solve problems in one area have affected other areas adversely. The credo to "do no harm" is often abused in health care and in national policy.

It's time to develop a vision and a direction. Insight, integrity and intelligence are needed.

What can be done to promote wellness and wholeness for people of all sizes? Critical challenges need to be addressed in the areas of attitude, lifestyle, health care, prevention, and knowledge.

1. Attitude

The attitude challenge is to develop a wider awareness and concern for the issues of weight, among both health professionals and the general public. Further, we each need to develop positive attitudes toward the pleasurable and beneficial aspects of healthy lifestyles. Needs in meeting the attitude challenge:

- **Accept a wider range of shapes and sizes:** appreciate diversity and individual differences in others; confront size discrimination when found; enhance self-acceptance and positive self-image; end body hatred.

- **Change media and advertising focus or influence:** decrease the obsession with thinness in the media and advertising; encourage media portrayal of healthy lifestyles for children and adults; issue complaints

Beauty ideas are fluid

African American girls hold flexible and fluid images of beauty in contrast to rigid and fixed images held by white girls, in a University of Arizona study of 300 adolescent girls.

Nearly three-fourths of the African American girls were satisfied with their weight, despite the fact that many were significantly overweight. Beauty for them was not related to size, but to "looking good." This meant projecting their self-image and confidence, establishing a presence, creating and presenting a sense of style, and "making what you have work for you."

In contrast, most white girls were dissatisfied with their bodies and wanted to lose weight as a way to be popular and "perfect." Over 90 percent were dissatisfied with their weight, even when normal.

They struggled to achieve a specific standard of body size and beauty. "Indeed, their ideal girl was described with striking uniformity: she was about 5'7", 120 pounds, had long blonde hair and long, long legs. When girls compared themselves to this ideal, it led to a devaluation of their own looks and a sense of personal dissatisfaction and frustration. The notion of an ideal, perfect girl was particularly salient during early adolescence," said the report.

Other white girls expressed envy and competitiveness for girls who came closest to this ideal, unlike African American girls, who described themselves as supportive of each other. They told of positive feedback from family, friends and community about "looking good."

The researchers suggest these flexible attitudes about beauty need to be supported, explored and encouraged among the white girls.[51]

or boycott thin stereotyping in magazines, TV and advertising; teach evaluation of advertising in schools at preadolescent levels; regulate advertising of high fat and high sugar foods to children.

- **Appreciate the importance of healthy lifestyles:** focus on the pleasurable and beneficial effects of healthy lifestyle patterns, not on size, shape or weight.

- **Understand the issues of weight:** learn and teach the importance of preventing obesity and disordered eating in both children and adults, the risks of weight loss practices; the difficulty of losing weight in a lasting way, the benefits of maintaining a stable weight; also the harmful effects of childhood sexual abuse and its relation to disordered eating.

The body cannot be shaped at will, individual differences in body shapes and sizes are natural and desirable.

The values of tolerance, respect, and appreciation of diversity need to be taught and modeled by parents, educators and health policy makers. People need to understand that the body cannot be shaped at will, that individual differences in body shapes and sizes are natural and desirable.

Body images are severe for young people today, particularly for adolescent girls. If they are to develop into strong, competent, caring women, it can be extremely harmful for them to idealize female images which are emaciated, vulnerable, passive and childlike.

An Arizona study that compared ideals of beauty between white adolescent girls and African American girls shows a clear contrast between healthy and unhealthy attitudes.

The African American girls' images of beauty were found to be flexible, fluid, not related to a particular size or ideal. They were based on each girl's sense of self and style, her confidence, and "looking good." She was supported in this by other girls and by family, friends and community.

Sadly, the images held by white girls in this study are painful in contrast. Their ideal was narrow, rigid and, for most, unattainable. Almost as one they described their "perfect girl." She weighed 120 pounds, and had very long legs and long blonde hair. Comparing themselves to this ideal, the girls were dissatisfied with their weight and appearance. Nearly all wanted to lose weight as a way to "be perfect" and popular. Perversely, the girls did not support those among them who were closest to this ideal, but rather expressed envy and competitiveness. The younger girls in early adolescence were most severely affected by these self-defeating images.[1]

The African American girls attitudes are supportive of a healthy body image and positive self-esteem. Yet this example raises immediate concerns among some health policy makers: Will self-acceptance by teenage girls cause them to relax their vigilance, let themselves go, and gain too much weight? Wouldn't it be better if the African American girls (who may be more susceptible to weight gain) began to fear for their figures, were less accepting, and learned to restrain eating?

The answer is not more fear, but less. Solutions must be found that support size acceptance, while at the same time reducing the prevalence of obesity in indirect ways through healthy lifestyle patterns. The recent rise in obesity rates is a serious concern; however it must be dealt with in ways that "do no harm."

Clearly it is a national crisis when harmful attempts at dieting are common in the third grade, when more than two-thirds of high school girls are dieting, one in five have taken diet pills, and many girls as well as boys are using laxatives, diuretics, fasting and vomiting in frantic attempts to trim their bodies down as thin as possible.

This is the point where extremely thin ideals have brought us in a culture obsessed with weight. This is truly a crime against our children. Children are the innocent victims.

Efforts like the national "Women's Campaign to End Body Hatred and Dieting," sponsored by the National Center for Overcoming Overeating, directed by Carol Munter and Jane Hirschmann, and "International No Diet Day," on May 6, are aimed at changing attitudes about weight which have been especially detrimental to women.

It is important that women be portrayed in the media as real people of varied shapes, sizes and talents, deserving of respect. Today's typical media images of women – as decorative or sexual objects to be admired or used – need to be discouraged. Women are not objects or toys, and it is most unfortunate when pre-adolescent girls are led to believe that they should fill these roles. As women move into decision-making positions this situation improves, therefore it is imperative to speed this process.

The media and advertisers need to be enlisted in helping people appreciate diversity by portraying a wider range of sizes and shapes. It seems possible that if only two or three teen magazines and women's magazines had the courage to depict women of all sizes in their pages, the entire focus of the thin cultural stereotype would begin to change. Other editors and television producers might suddenly discover the beauty, charm and unique talents of real women in all their diversity.

Today only a very few dare to break through the tyranny of portraying women as a single thin stereotype. Three companies that have were honored during 1995 Healthy Weight Week (the third week in January) for their national leadership portraying people, especially women, of a diversity of sizes. Selected as leaders in this were CNN television network, Wal-Mart stores and Snapple beverage company.

Consumers groups, too, can make a difference. BAM (Boycott Anorexic Marketing), a Boston-based consumer group, boycotted Diet Sprite and forced the company to drop an offensive ad that depicted a bony, apathetic girl sipping a diet drink, while boasting of her nickname "Skeleton."

Schools need to teach the power of advertising and how to protect one's self-image from narrow media stereotypes, beginning in pre-adolescence where media images have perhaps their greatest impact. Children can understand that many advertisers focus on extremes to make their products seem "even more so" than similar products – i.e. "if long legs are good, our models have longer legs than anyone else's; if wide-spaced eyes and hollow cheeks are attractive, ours are spaced even wider, our cheeks more gaunt."

It is also important for health care providers and the lay public to better understand the perspective of large persons. Many large individuals are silent in the face of extreme criticism and prejudice. This may be taken for agreement but may mask a sense of helplessness, resentment and rage. Activists in the size acceptance movement are bringing these issues into the open, and educators, health care providers, and state and

Boost self-esteem with fat affirmations
by Karen W. Stimson

Affirmations can create a new vision for ourselves and point us in the direction we want to go. They can help us to quiet the self-depreciating voices we carry inside.

1. I am a beautiful fat woman/man, with unique talents and abilities, and I am worthy of self-respect and the respect of others.
2. I feel good/I am learning to feel good about myself today, accept my body the size and shape it is now, and love myself.
3. I do not/I am learning not to compare my size or shape to anyone else's, to any standards.
4. I listen/I am learning to listen to what my body tells me about hunger and fullness, and I give myself permission to eat as much of whatever foods I want.
5. I give myself/I am learning to give myself permission to take up as much space as my body needs.
6. I expect/I am learning to expect to be treated with respect at all times and strive to project a positive self-image.
7. I do not give any person or institution permission to discriminate against me in any way or to make me feel bad.
8. I refuse/I am learning to refuse to be victimized or demeaned.
9. I react/I am learning to react to incidents of discrimination, whether directed at me or at other fat people, in ways that empower us, both politically and personally.[52]
Reprinted from NAAFA News, March 1992.

Schools need to focus more on helping all youngsters be physically active in ways that will last a lifetime, and less on star athletes and winning games.

national leaders would do well to listen with an open mind. These leaders need to recognize that they are often considered to be part of an insensitive, paternalistic power structure which causes much oppression.

Finally, people need to feel encouraged to make healthy changes in their own lives. They need to believe they can fit physical activity and other beneficial lifestyle patterns into their everyday lives in ways that are enjoyable. Motivational messages need to come from schools, health care providers, parents, peers and the media.

2. Lifestyle

An urgent challenge is to improve what has been called the unhealthy American lifestyle. We need to redouble efforts to help people of all ages develop and enjoy lasting healthy lifestyle patterns including:

- **Being physically active.**
- **Eating moderately of a balanced, moderately low-fat diet:** eating normally, without dieting; stopping ineffective, unsafe dieting practices.
- **Keeping a stable weight:** not gaining weight or focusing on weight loss.
- **Reducing or managing stress:** enriching self-esteem and self-acceptance; interacting positively with family, friends and community; focusing on balance and moderation, not extremes, especially in exercise, eating and weight issues.
- **Establishing an environment that supports healthy lifestyles:** changing factors that lead to inactivity, overeating or increased stress; providing preventive and counseling programs for sexual abuse and violence against women.

Healthy lifestyle patterns need to be promoted in schools, health care settings, the community and the home, and through the media. Family influence is important. Parents and people of all ages can set good examples and improve their own health by making positive changes in gradual ways.

Most Americans urgently need to be more physically active. A nationwide public health program to encourage exercise is long overdue. Elsewhere such programs have long been active. The Council of Europe in 1966 adopted the longterm objective of "Sport for all." The Australian program "Life be in it!" went nationwide to encourage active living in 1977.

Communities can do much to encourage active living: developing safe, well-lighted playgrounds, parks, swimming pools, skating rinks, and trails for walking, bicycling and cross-country skiing. They can open school gymnasiums to the public, provide recreation centers, and organize fitness campaigns and events. At the national level, health policy makers should expand their efforts to advocate the pleasures and health benefits of an active lifestyle, especially for children, adolescents, the elderly and lower socioeconomic populations.

Physical education in schools needs to focus more on helping all youngsters be physically active in ways that will last a lifetime, and less on winning games, and grooming star athletes. Less emphasis on spectator sports and more on being personally involved would be helpful. Daily aerobic exercise should be required for children from kindergarten through high school, with a focus on fun and creativity, not competition. Competition isolates and discriminates against large and less fit children and discourages them from being active. The roadblocks that still keep many girls and women from being active in sports need to be removed, and active sports encouraged for all.

Most Americans are still eating too much fat. It is a personal responsibility to purchase less fat at the grocery, prepare foods with less fat, and add less fat at the table. Schools lunch programs are responding by serving less fat.

The food industry needs to include less fat in staple products: at restaurants, in processed foods, and at the meat counter. Changing federal regulations can make a difference, as in the amount of fat specified in hamburger and ice cream, and standards for agricultural products.

However, extremes should be avoided, and moderation encouraged. Eating should be a pleasurable experience. Unfortunately, advice to lower fat intake is being taken to ridiculous extremes by some people, to the extent of depriving small children of needed fat and calories for growth and development. About 25 to 30 percent fat is considered about right.

Eating smaller quantities may also be desirable. Observers say restaurants are increasing the size of their servings as they increase prices. Buffets which promote "all you can eat" may cause problems when indulged too frequently; even laboratory rats eat more when their food comes "cafeteria style."

3. Health care

A fresh approach for the health enhancement of persons with weight related problems is much needed, as well as earlier identification and treatment for disordered eating.

Health care needs:

■ **Focus on health, not weight loss, for large patients:** emphasize improved health; do not put a large child on a diet, which will rarely succeed, but use indirect, non-depriving ways of changing lifestyle patterns and increase activity levels in non-threatening, non-competitive, enjoyable environments; require that all weight loss treatments be proven safe and longterm effective before being used; encourage keeping a stable weight; understand that weight loss goals may not be appropriate and can cause harm; create a medical specialty to deal with obesity in an integrated way; follow the credo, "do no harm."

■ **Reduce size prejudice in health care:** be sensitive to large patients and treat them with respect; weigh only if necessary and in private; provide adequate accommodations.

■ **Treat disordered eating at early stage:** identify and help students with disordered eating; develop treatment programs for "chronic dieting syndrome" (frequent dieting followed by compulsive eating).

■ **Improve access to qualified services for high risk populations:** minorities, low income groups and children.

■ **Develop sound policy on drug treatment:** require longterm drug use to be established as safe and effective before advocated; begin dialogue on ethical decisions for future drug use.

■ **Require nutrition studies in medical schools:** expand medical training to include nutrition, obesity and eating studies (or teach students to refer to specialists).

■ **Regulate weight loss industry:** require reporting of adverse effects, morbidity and mortality; require safety and effectiveness studies; require program data and results.

Programs for large people need to focus on improved health and the prevention of further weight gain, rather than weight loss, which has not been successful. There is much evidence it is beneficial to maintain a stable weight, and therefore, weight loss goals may not be appropriate. "Do no harm" needs to be a credo everywhere, as in Canada, where physicians responded quickly to the national warning by modifying their weight-related advice.

Focus of treatment should be on the total person: developing or reinforcing healthy lifestyle patterns, enhancing self-esteem, learning assertive skills, coping with family and community life, developing each person's potential as a loveable, capable and worthwhile individual.

Many health care professionals are in the process of change, moving toward a health promotion model, and away from a weight loss focus.

Momentum is growing for the new, more open, nondiet programs led by nutritionists such as Ellyn Satter, MS, RD, Madison, Wis. *(How to Get your Kid to Eat – But Not Too Much)*, Linda Omichinski, RD, Winnipeg, Canada *(You Count, Calories Don't*, and *Hugs Facilitator Kit* program for leaders), Dayle Hayes, RD, Billings, Mont. *(Body Trust)*, Joanne Ikeda, MA, RD, Berkeley, Calif. *(If My Child is too Fat, What Should I Do?)*. These specialists and other leaders in nutrition, public health and eating disorder fields don't agree on all points. But they speak with clear, informed voices to issues on which the nation has been silent.

Health care providers need to be aware of their own weight-related issues and overcome prejudices. Many large persons avoid doctors due to a history of negative experiences in health care. Often they delay needed treatment while conditions worsen. Certainly they need to be treated with respect, tact and concern.

The weight loss business is a health care industry. It needs to be officially regarded as such, and held accountable as other health care providers. Requirements for full disclosure of adverse effects and tracking of program effectiveness are needed. New York City and New York State are leaders in setting standards which may be useful as model legislation elsewhere.

Regulatory agencies have been more diligent in enforcing deceptive advertising and anti-fraud laws since the 1990 congressional hearings. The Federal Trade Commission has been especially active in pressing charges against illegal weight loss advertising. This needs to continue.

The current promotion of longterm drug treatment for obesity by many health authorities is cause for concern. Safety and effectiveness have not been established, and the potential for abuse is high. Even health officials who promote wider drug use for the treatment of obesity agree there is "insufficient research" for this, and that "longterm studies are warranted."[2]

The medical community has allowed the abuse of other medications, so excessive misuse can be expected, warns Joe McVoy, PhD, an eating disorder specialist in Virginia. "Millions of men and women will again be asked to begin long term treatment before proof of its safety or

Editors and television producers might suddenly discover the beauty, charm and unique talents of real women in all their diversity.

effectiveness are established."

Other concerns are how drugs will be used, and by whom? When safe and effective drugs are available, perhaps in 10 to 15 years, will they be marketed to children? It's time to begin the dialogue on ethical decisions for future use of these drugs.

4. Prevention

Prevention efforts should have the three goals of (1) improving lifestyle habits for people of all ages, (2) decreasing dieting behavior and eating disorders, with special concern for children and adolescent girls, and (3) the prevention of excess weight gain, especially for high-risk populations – minorities, low-income groups, and women.
Needs are to:

- **Encourage healthy lifestyles:** promote physical activity, stress reduction, good nutrition and normal eating for people of all ages, through the environment, media, schools, community; improve the environment through the food industry, federal agencies, schools, community and family.

- **Initiate effective prevention programs:** research, develop, test and implement programs to prevent obesity and disordered eating, evaluating to ensure they do no harm; require early preventive education in schools; increase research to identify and help persons at high risk for obesity.

Among the many ironies and difficulties in the weight field are that when obesity risks and the need for action on this front are emphasized, so are the fear of fat and the disordered eating pressures which go with it. All too easily, we foster thin mania, eating disorders, size-oppression, social and economic discrimination, and an increase in hazardous weight loss products and services. Risk of intensifying the existing problems is even more acute when we deal with the vulnerability of children. The wrong kind of intervention is often worse than excess weight.

For these reasons it is critical that prevention programs be carefully researched and found both safe and effective before being widely implemented. The nationwide lack of interest in prevention by the medical community and public health has been disappointing. Americans have long put their faith in magic bullets. In weight issues it is clear that the real magic bullet is prevention.

Healthy lifestyle habits are considered preventive of both obesity and eating disorders. Healthy changes in these areas can do much to prevent both these problems and should be the initial focus. Encouraging physical activity, promoting safe biking and hiking trails, swimming pools, basketball courts, and participation in sports for all is important. The national Canadian *Vitality* program is of this type, encouraging healthy activity, eating well and feeling good about oneself.

However, the problems are so acute in the U.S. today that these are not likely to be enough. Research and new knowledge for initiating safe and effective preventive programs are urgently needed.

In obesity, the primary aim should be to reduce the number of new cases of obesity and to limit further weight gain in large persons. Another aim may be to delay the onset of obesity, which may reduce its duration and severity.

Research needs to find successful ways to target high risk individu-

Preventing eating disorders in Norway

Norway is one of the first countries to launch an eating disorder prevention program, with the Eating Disorders Project which began in 1993 in a one county pilot program.

Focus is on education of all youngsters through the schools, coupled with early intervention for students with disordered eating, and longterm active treatment for serious eating disorders. Support groups will be formed, and eating disorder treatment centers will be evaluated for effectiveness.

Manuals were developed, and training held for school nurses and teachers, with special emphasis on coaches and trainers, since athletes are considered at special risk. Of Norwegian female elite athletes, 18 percent have serious eating disorders. Many reported that coaches' criticism or demands to reduce weights led to their eating problems. In the pilot county 5 percent of students, age 12 to 19, were identified as having eating disorders, an estimated 40,000 throughout Norway.

Research on effectiveness will compare 1,000 ninth graders in the pilot schools with control children from another county. The prevention program is expected to have a positive effect on lowering the incidence of eating disorders, as well as shortening treatment for diagnosed patients, due to earlier intervention.

The socialized nature of the Norwegian health care system makes eating disorders treatment a public responsibility, resulting in strong support for prevention efforts.[54]

10 things men can do and be to help prevent eating disorders

by Michael P. Levine, PhD

1. Reject the notion that eating disorders are a women's issue. In the 1890s and 1920s, and since 1970, eating disorders have flourished in an atmosphere of anxiety and anger about women's rights and opportunities. Thus, eating disorders are, in a very important sense, sociopolitical issues with a clear connection to men and power.

2. Think seriously and constantly about yourself as a gendered being. Consider, for example, how free and independent you really are when you hesitate before putting on an apron or buying tampons; or when you reflexively consider shooting baskets and talking with a friend to be a waste of time, as opposed to playing one-on-one.

3. Take your role as a father, brother and/or uncle seriously. Men play a very significant role in the emotional and psychosocial development of girls and boys. Abnegation of the role of father, in particular, in the name of work or success or lack of time is a contribution to (a) the emotional distress ("hunger") underlying eating disorders in females; and (b) feelings of powerlessness, insecurity and rage in males that fuel the oppression of women through objectification, pornography and other forms of violence.

4. Accept responsibility for learning about sexism within our patriarchal and capitalist society. Feminists are tired, and justifiably so, of repeatedly explaining to well-meaning but ultimately conde- scending males what feminism is all about.

5. Abandon sexism. Sexism offers men the promise of privilege, influence, and control, but at the expense of both our relationships with others (men and women) and our self-development through caring, feeling, sensitivity and equality.

6. Accept the notion that men must change themselves and other men (including sons). Too many changes have been required of women already, and the resulting stress and role confusion most certainly contributes to disordered eating. Changes by and in men, while initially difficult, will ultimately benefit both sexes.

7. Don't just acknowledge conflict for women in changing gender roles, experience it for yourself. Start by endeavoring to be a person instead of a "success object."

8. Take personal and political action against sexism. Men can contribute to the prevention of eating disorders by changing their own behavior and/or the behavior of others so as to:
(a) reverse discrimination against girls and women in school, in the workplace, on the streets, and at home;
(b) ensure that women are free from harassment, sexual abuse, physical intimidation and other forms of violence to their bodies and souls;
(c) encourage women (and men) to accept and develop themselves as people, not as attractive packages based on restrictive ideals of beauty and self-restraint;
(d) develop relationships between (and images of) men and women based on respect, not exploitation.

9. Give positive messages. What messages on glorifying slenderness and vilifying body fat do you intentionally or inadvertently communicate to the men/boys and girls/women in your life? Educate yourself, your children, your students, about:
(a) the genetic basis of differences in body types;
(b) media manipulation of ideal body types and body dissatisfaction;
(c) the nature and ugliness of prejudice against fat people;
(d) the dangers of restrictive dieting and weight cycling.

10. Listen to women. Spend lots of time being silent and listening (really listening) to what women have to say. As immortalized in the work of Carl Rogers, authentic respect in the form of nonjudgmental listening can be truly empowering (whereas a successful diet cannot).[3]

Reprinted with permission. Adapted with minor revisions from an article in the Newsletter of the National Eating Disorders Organization (NEDO), April-May 1994. The author thanks Linda Smolak, PhD (Kenyon College), and Barbara Carney (Bulimia Anorexia Nervosa Association, Canada) for their feedback. Michael Levine, PhD, is Professor of Psychology at Kenyon College, Gambier, OH and an educational consultant to NEDO.

als and groups, such as children of obese parents, and women during critical life events – adolescence, pregnancy and menopause. Populations undergoing sudden cultural change are also at risk, but there's still time to do much prevention in places like Alaska, and the Pacific Islands.

Although obesity has received most attention in the U.S., the prevention of eating disorders is equally important and needs to be regarded seriously by the medical community.

Norway has established a comprehensive program of eating disorders prevention which focuses on three areas: education of all youngsters through the schools; early intervention for disordered eating; and longterm active treatment for people with eating disorders. Upcoming research on the effectiveness of the program will be valuable for use elsewhere.

5. Knowledge

Weight research is a relatively young science and offers many knowledge challenges:

■ **Increase research and understanding:** more research is needed on the causes, treatment and prevention of obesity: how the fat cell stores and protects fat, body regulation of weight, appetite, satiety, and hunger, prevention and treatment of eating disorders, the physical and mental effects of starvation, and the nature of the "thrifty gene" that increases obesity for populations undergoing sudden cultural change.

■ **Communicate knowledge:** provide wider access to understanding on weight issues to professionals and the lay public; increase the impact of women's research, particularly as it affects women's issues related to weight and eating disorders; gain more access for women scientists in conference reporting and scientific publishing.

■ **Consolidate weight studies:** bring together research, education and communication within one discipline, with close networking between related fields.

■ **Raise ethical standards:** of scientific conferences, journals, organizations, and health care policies in this field which may be unduly influenced by vested interests.

We need to know a great deal more about the causes, nature, treatment and prevention of obesity. What are the genetic and environmental factors and how are they interrelated? The challenge is to increase the understanding of weight issues and disseminate both information and understanding among health care professionals, educators and consumers.

Research by women needs to be reported more widely in conferences and in the scientific press. The almost total domination by males in research, publishing and health care decisions has slowed recognition of the importance of women's issues in obesity and eating disorders. Women scientists still struggle to get their work accepted. Sexual bias affects scientific conferences, organizations, publications and health care.

In late 1994, prominent female obesity researchers filed a complaint with organizers of the 7th International Congress on Obesity in Toronto charging that all plenary speakers were men and only 10 percent of other invited segments of the meeting were women, even though one-third of attendees were women. This lack, the complaint said, "is not only glaring,

> *"It is almost impossible to find any boundary between government, industry and the medical elite . . . It is a tightly interlocking system that would make apologists for the military-industrial complex blush."*
> – Thomas Moore

but unjustifiable."

Ethics in the treatment field is another serious problem which needs to be aired. Obesity research has been particularly vulnerable to the power of vested interests.

Thomas Moore, of George Washington University, in his book *Lifespan: Who Lives Longer and Why?,* speaks directly to this problem. "It is almost impossible to find any boundary between the government, the industry and the medical elite . . . It is a closed circle of medical insiders operating without the normal checks and ethical barriers . . . a tightly interlocking system that would make apologists for the military-industrial complex blush," said Moore.

Presentations of industry-slanted research which manipulates the data, or evades or obscures the whole truth, or gives short-term, irrelevant findings as if they were lasting, should not be permitted during major sessions of scientific conferences. This is not science.

The use of public funds or public institutions for this kind of pseudoscience should be discouraged.

Finally, weight studies need to be brought together within one discipline so the information can be researched, analyzed and used in a comprehensive way, while networking with other closely related fields. Nutrition would seem the logical choice for consolidating these studies, since it has great depth in most of the relevant areas, including both obesity and eating disorders.

Male domination in research, has slowed recognition of the importance of women's issues in obesity and eating disorders.

Healthy decisions

These are complex and controversial issues. They need to be dealt with wisely and sensitively, with an understanding of the critical health issues involved. Women and children's concerns need to be carefully considered.

It's time to develop a vision and direction. These are critical and urgent challenges for this nation.

The process of developing a unified vision of where we are and where we want to go will ideally involve ordinary citizens representing many points of view, educators in community and kindergarten through graduate school, health care providers, public policy makers and specialists in related fields.

It's important that decision makers be people of insight, intelligence and integrity. They must be people who are willing to consider other's viewpoints and able to understand what is happening all across the weight spectrum. We can no longer permit these critical decisions to be made by people who refuse to consider the effect their decisions may have on women and on persons of all sizes, or who serve the weight loss industry.

We need to deal with this weight crisis in healthy ways – ways that don't repeat the mistakes of the past.

APPENDIX

Obesity definitions

For purposes of this report, *obesity* is defined in a general way as any degree of excess weight or body fat. The terms *overweight* and *large* are also used in this generic sense, interchangeably with *obese.*

Most researchers and educators appear to be using the terms *obese* and *obesity* in this general way. However, U.S. health publications use the term *overweight,* to denote any degree of excess weight or fat, avoiding *obesity* as being more objectionable to consumers, and with the explanation that weight (not fat) is the criteria normally used in research.

A single precise definition of obesity has not yet been determined. Obesity is defined in various ways as follows:

1. Obesity as any degree of excess weight or fat

Obesity can be used in a general way to denote any degree of excess weight or fat over a designated level, according to height/weight tables or body mass index (BMI), which is also based on height and weight. Frequent cut-off points are 120 percent of so-called *ideal* weight, or BMI of 25 or 27. (The National Center for Health Statistics uses BMI of 27.8 or more for men and 27.3 or more for women, reported to be about 124 percent of *desirable* for men and 120 percent of *desirable* for women.)

2. Obesity as the highest of three weight categories

Some researchers use the three categories *ideal weight, overweight and obesity.* In this definition, overweight may be 110-119 percent of the *ideal* range; obesity 120 percent or more. Or obesity may refer to a BMI of 30 or more; overweight, 25 to 30. This definition was common in the past, but is used less today by researchers.

3. Obesity as excessive body fat

Many hold that this is the correct definition, that *obesity* should be defined in terms of excess body fat. Body fat can be independent of weight, so in theory an obese person may not be overweight, and vice versa. However, in practice, even when obesity is defined as excess fat in this way, it is usually measured in terms of weight, so at this time the definition seems impractical.

4. Obesity as the level at which health risk begins

An ideal definition, some experts say, would be to define obesity as the point above which either excess weight or fat contributes to an increase in risk factors related to obesity. Two problems exist with this. First, this point is currently unknown, and when it is, will probably differ for individuals as related to factors such as genetics, fat distribution, dieting history, lifestyle and physical activity. Second, there are certain areas in which health is not a factor at all, such as social and political issues.

Note: O*besity* and *obese* are far from satisfactory terms, and other terms are equally unsatisfactory. The Latin root of *obesity* is *to eat,* and thus the word does not convey its complex causes. The development of better semantics is a need in this field. (From a consumer point of view the word *obese* is unsatisficatory, having unpleasant connotations. It is recommended that *obese* be used only as an adjective, not as a noun, and that the term *severe obesity* be used rather than *morbid obesity.*)

1992 NIH conference statement

The National Institutes of Health Technology Assessment on Methods for Voluntary Weight Loss and Control Conference was held March 30–April 1, 1992. Following are excerpts from the conference statement.

A health paradox exists in modern America. On the one hand, many people who do not need to lose weight are trying to. On the other hand, most who do need to lose weight are not succeeding. The percentage of Americans whose health is jeopardized by too much weight is increasing. Thus, consideration of voluntary weight loss must encompass a continuum from persons of normal or low weight who wish to lose weight for cultural, social, or psychological reasons to severely overweight persons who suffer clear adverse medical consequences.

Approximately one quarter to one third of adults in the United States are classified as overweight, depending on the BMI cut point used. The prevalence has increased during the last two decades. The prevalence is disproportionately high in many populations, especially in women, the poor, and members of some ethnic groups.

Being overweight can seriously affect health and longevity. It is associated with elevated serum cholesterol, elevated blood pressure, and noninsulin-dependent diabetes mellitus. Excessive weight also increases the risk for gallbladder disease, gout, coronary heart disease, and some types of cancer and has been implicated in the development of osteoarthritis of the weight-bearing joints.

Although there seems to be little doubt that overweight individuals have increased risk for morbidity and mortality, it does not immediately follow that weight loss reduces that increased risk.

In controlled settings, diets, behavior modification, exercise, and drugs produce short-term weight losses with reasonable safety. Unfortunately, most people who achieve weight loss with any of these programs regain weight.

Successful weight loss improves control of noninsulin-dependent diabetes mellitus and hypertension, reduces cardiovascular risk factors, and enhances self-image. Long-term health effects are much less clear.

Given the high likelihood that weight will be regained, it remains to be determined whether these time-limited improvements confer more permanent health benefits.

Understanding the health consequences of weight loss requires data on what happens to those who have lost weight. For most weight loss methods, there are few scientific studies evaluating their effectiveness and safety. The available studies indicate that persons lose weight in such programs but, after completing the program, tend to regain the weight over time.

Further, there are examples where weight loss strategies have caused medical harm. Thus, the panel cautions that before individuals adopt any weight loss program, the scientific data on effectiveness and safety be examined. If no data exist, the panel recommends that the program not be used. The lack of data on many commercial programs advertised for weight loss is especially disconcerting in view of the large number of Americans trying to lose weight and the over $30 billion spent yearly in America on weight loss efforts.

Data on short-term adverse health effects of weight loss come from programs that only include overweight persons. Some of these effects may be greater in persons who are not overweight but are severely restricting calories. Laboratory evidence suggests that weight loss in lean persons leads to a greater proportional loss of lean body mass than in severely overweight persons.

The fact that many adolescents and young adults use over-the-counter preparations urges further study of their safety in real-world use. Although currently used weight-reducing drugs appear to be safe in controlled studies, (they) are short term and have involved populations where potential for abuse may be low.

Participants in formal weight loss programs may reduce baseline depression and anxiety, but only if they successfully lose weight. Little is known about the emotional impact of lesser degrees of success or of failure. There also is increasing evidence that mildly to moderately overweight women who are dieting may be at risk for binge-eating.

Several epidemiologic studies raise the possibility that weight loss is associated with increased mortality. (However), in most of these studies the reason for weight loss is not known. Intentional weight loss during healthy states cannot be distinguished from that associated with illness, psychosocial distress, or other reasons. Finally, the fact that many people who stop smoking gain weight complicates the interpretation of the data on weight gainers and weight losers. Thus, although the data on higher mortality are provocative, they are not sufficiently conclusive to dictate clinical practice. Specific research efforts to address this question are urgently needed.

New York City investigation

The New York City Department of Consumer Affairs (DCA) investigated segments of the weight loss industry and released the report A Weighty Issue: Dangers and Deceptions of the Weight Loss Industry in June 1991. Below are excerpts from this report.

Weight loss centers are big business, generating more than $2.3 billion in total sales, and annually catering to about two million people. There are at least nine major weight loss services with scores of branches in the New York metropolitan region. (Weight Watchers, Optifast; Medifast; Diet Center; United Weight Control; Nutri/System; Herbal Life; Dick Gregory Bahamian Diet; Slim Time Weight Loss Center.)

There are currently no federal regulations to oversee the maze of diet programs out on the market, nor are there any minimum standards for operating such programs. Consumers often mistakenly believe that diet clinics are licensed, but, in fact, they are not regulated by any state or local authority.

The huge growth of this unregulated industry in the past decade and the rising tide of questionable practices regarding these services prompted Congressional hearings last year by Rep. Ron Wyden (D.-Ore.), chairman of the House Subcommittee on Regulation, Business Opportunities and Energy. Wyden warned: "Most commercial clinics promise fast, safe, easy weight loss. Most experts agree that fast weight loss is dangerous in and of itself. Further, little research has been done to show what does and does not work for each individual."

In 1989, a special Task Force assembled by the Michigan Health Council warned that the weight loss industry was placing citizens at significant health risk.

Investigating 3 segments

The Consumer Affairs researched three segments of the commercial weight loss industry:

- Rapid weight loss programs in which the person fasts on liquid formula, supposedly supervised by physicians and hospitals.
- Commercial weight loss centers that restrict the diet through regimented meal plans.
- Commercial meal-replacement powders.

There is huge competition for patient dollars between these rival approaches and companies. At their height in 1989, the manufacturers of Optifast and HMR – two physician-sponsored liquid formula programs – were taking in a combined $600 million a year, controlling about 75 percent of that market.

Since the late 1980s, however, sales have been climbing for over-the-counter diet powders.

In addition to drawing sheer numbers, these programs have been assured the golden opportunity of repeat sales – virtually guaranteed precisely because the majority of dieters don't keep off the weight. Chronic dieters invariably try more than one program.

DCA staff, posing as potential clients, called or visited 14 weight loss centers that restrict diet. We found:

- Nine out of ten surveyed centers did not give advance warning or openly discuss the potential safety risks involved in their specific program or of rapid weight loss in general, even when directly asked about possible health problems.
- Some weight loss centers attempted to sell their weight loss services to people who did not need them – including the underweight. (One underweight woman was told she could lose five pounds, which would have put her statistically at risk for certain medical problems.)
- Some centers are engaged more in quackery than medicine. At one clinic we were told that gorging on certain foods could speed up metabolism.
- Some weight loss centers subject prospective customers to high pressure sales tactics that verge on harassment.

Health hazards

The low calorie regimens can cause potentially serious health hazards and weight loss centers fail to explicitly warn potential customers of these hazards. Over-the-counter meal-replacement powders fail to warn that misusing the product can be hazardous to one's health or possibly even fatal.

Thirty-four million people nationwide are more than 20 percent over their ideal weight. This medical problem is linked to many potential health risks that can lead to stroke, heart disease and diabetes. But what is less known to consumers is that the treatment of obesity can also result in heart injury, gallbladder injury, and a host of other serious conditions.

There had been particular concern with losing weight rapidly on liquid formula diets, which have seen a popular resurgence in recent years. In such diets, a woman typically loses 3 pounds a week and a man 5 pounds a week, cutting their calories to under

800 a day. In the most extreme low calorie diets, the person receives about 400 calories a day, usually in the form of a powdered drink, which is supervised by a doctor who typically monitors the patient once a week.

Weight loss occurs when the output of energy expended by the body exceeds the number of calories the person has available from food. The body uses its own fat reserves, but if weight loss is too rapid, the body will also draw from lean mass; when this happens, muscle and organ tissue is gradually lost. This loss can include the heart, which is a muscle.

President of the American Dietetic Association Dr. Nancy Wellman, warns that, "the most significant drawback to these diets is the potential for life-threatening side effects. The loss of body protein – and here we are talking about muscle tissue – may affect cardiac function and could be related to heart failure."

The health risks associated with low calorie diets have been the subject of debate since the 1970s, after 58 people suddenly diet while fasting on liquid formula diets, such as the well-known Cambridge diet. While medical experts agree that current formula diets are better than the old formulas, what the diet companies themselves do know is that health complications if not fatalities are possible with their diets.

It is impossible, however, to know if sudden deaths are still occurring since there is currently no mechanism for tracking diet-related deaths.

United Weight Control Corp., a medically-supervised fasting program affiliated with St. Lukes/Roosevelt Hospital Center in Manhattan, spells out the dangers in the tiny type of an "Informed Consent for Treatment" contract that dieters sign when they embark on the program. It reads:

"Some reports have suggested a relationship between programmed diets and sudden death, probably due to irregularities of the heart. I understand that participation in this weight reduction program may entail a minute risk of fatal heart irregularities."

Although weight loss centers know of the health risks associated with major weight loss, they typically do not warn the person in advance or openly discuss the dangers with potential customers.

Gallstones form

About 30 New York diet victims (are) alleging severe gallbladder injuries from the Nutri/System diet; 25 New Yorkers are suing the company . . . In Florida, 72 cases have been filed against Nutri/System, with 100 additional cases due to be filed, all from people on the program who developed severe gallbladder injuries.

In the wake of the bad publicity, Nutri/System

replied to the gallbladder injury cases in a series of ads last year that state: "Obesity – not dieting – is a major cause of gallbladder disease."

While it is true that obese people are prone to developing gallstones, there are published studies showing that dieters develop gallstones on diets. According to Dr. C. Wayne Callaway, Associate Clinical Professor of Medicine at George Washington University, "Heavier people have more cholesterol in their bile. With dieting, the bile acid concentration goes down which allows cholesterol to form stones."

"The reasons for dieters developing gallstones is not yet fully understood and more research is needed," according to Dr. Xavier Pi-Sunyer, director of the Obesity Research Center at St. Lukes/Roosevelt Hospital Center in Manhattan. "There are some studies that suggest gallstones are more likely to form during the periods when you lose weight. There is also some evidence in the literature, although it's not conclusive, that the lower number of calories you're on, the more likely you'll develop gallstones."

In addition to the potential side effects already mentioned, rapid weight loss can also cause:
- Increased uric acid levels in the blood, which can cause or exacerbate gout or uric acid kidney stones
- Electrolyte imbalance: excessively low levels of potassium in the blood, which may lead to cardiac arrhythmias
- Anemia, characterized by fatigue, lassitude, weakness, pallor, reduced resistance to infection, lowered exercise tolerance and decreased attention span
- Fibrosis of vital organs: an abnormal increase in fibrous connective tissue in the organs may occur with repeated attempts at weight loss using starvation methods.
- Menstrual irregularities
- Constipation
- Dry skin
- Temporary skin rash
- Dizziness upon sudden standing
- Unusual pressure in the nerve of the leg which can lead to numbness or loss of muscle power
- Emotional stress, agitation, excessive anxiety or depression
- Overeating
- Dehydration
- Hair loss (usually temporary)
- Inability to maintain long-term weight loss.

Some people repeatedly lose and regain their weight, called "weight cycling" or the "yo yo syndrome." Medical authorities say that this can cause a persons's body to physiologically resist further weight loss. Despite the fact many chronic dieters suffer this fasting/feasting syndrome, no attempts have been made to discern the health risks attributed to obesity from those attributed to weight cycling.

While the range of services that diet programs offer varies, so do the experience and qualifications of the people who run them. In the liquid diet segment in those medically-supervised programs, the qualifications of the doctors may run the gamut of experience: some weight loss physicians are seasoned physicians with advanced training in nutrition while others may have only received rudimentary nutrition courses at a medical school. Some programs offer nutritional counseling by registered dietitians; others use nonprofessionals such as ex-clients.

Generally, people who sign up to slim down at a weight loss clinic are led to believe they are receiving a health-care service. But in such a commercially-driven atmosphere, too often the center's goal becomes sales, not health.

Even diet programs affiliated with physicians and hospitals may be more interested in generating profit than providing quality treatment. Psychiatrists have also gotten into the side-line business of putting patients on Medifast, another meal replacement fasting plan.

False claims

The drive to make sales may cause some companies to resort to making false claims. (The example is given of Stanford University's lawsuit against Nutri/System for false claims.)

Overweight people are susceptible to sales come-ons because many are often so desperate to lose weight.

The daily barrage of commercials and television shows emphasizing thinness as an ideal reinforces the message that overweight people don't fit into society. In their shame and embarrassment, many overweight people are driven into isolation. Their vulnerability makes them easy targets for diet services promising quick results and an end to their low self esteem. As Rep. Wyden warns, "Desperation for quick weight loss can cause consumers to make bad choices based on scant knowledge."

Our national preoccupation with maintaining the ideal body image obsesses even the bone-thin. Today fashion models are, on average, about 16 percent underweight.

Weight regain

Studies show that most dieters regain their weight. There is a lack of demonstrated long-term benefits of very low calorie diets. Sales representatives typically lead consumers to expect that their program will succeed on a long-term basis even if others have failed.

But in reality, no weight loss program can guarantee long-term success because programs do not monitor past clients on an ongoing basis. One may argue that keeping track of past clients isn't necessary; if the client faithfully follows the program, he or she will learn how to maintain their weight loss. But research shows that very low calorie diets fail because of the body's own physiological adaptation to a reduced caloric intake – not because the dieter returns to bad eating habits.

A plan for long-term maintenance is nearly always stressed by the weight loss centers. What is not discussed, however, is that studies have shown that the majority of overweight people who lose weight regain it back within a few years.

In studies of fat people who go on very low calorie diets, the results for long-term maintenance are very poor, according to Dr. Ernst Drenick, an obesity researcher with the Veterans Administration Medical Center in Loss Angeles, who tracked 100 morbidly obese men and found that nearly all regained their weight following a severe diet.

Weight loss centers often claim their success lies in helping the client change their behavior for life. They offer behavior modification classes to help the dieter learn, for example, what emotional cues trigger overeating.

But the fact remains: there are no long-term studies to back up the claim that behavior modification works over the long haul, according to the American Medical Association's Council on Scientific Affairs. The findings of one five-year follow-up of 36 individuals who participated in a behavioral program for obesity showed a typical pattern of regaining all the weight lost during treatment.

Diet programs will argue that their own studies show the weight loss is maintained. What the programs do not so readily indicate is that the studies are not long term. Most only gauge the dieter a year or less after the weight loss, according to Dr. Callaway.

Medical authorities say a year is not long enough to determine if the program has really worked or not, and may only indicate one phase in a weight cycling pattern.

Potential side effects of very low calorie diets

by the Michigan Health Council

Diets providing fewer than 800 calories per day have potential side effects which may vary with the person and composition of the diet. It is strongly recommended these diets be used only in a strictly supervised hospital setting, and only when the consequences of the obesity are a greater life threat than potential complications of low calorie intake.

■ **Cardiac arrhythmias:** Prolonged QT interval, ventricular fibrillation, multifocal premature ventricular contractions, and atrial fibrillation have all been observed. Arrhythmias can occur suddenly, without warning, and are potentially fatal.

■ **Inability to maintain long-term weight loss:** Rapid and/or repeated weight loss may slow basal metabolic rate, reducing calories needed. Lost weight may be regained quickly, and be more difficult to lose again in the future. Depression and diminished self-esteem are likely sequelae to weight regain.

■ **Initiation of binge eating:** The event initiating the development of anorexia and bulimia is almost invariably severe calorie restriction.

■ **Emotional changes:** VLCDs have been associated with emotional withdrawal, depression, anxiety and irritability.

■ **Loss of body protein:** Muscle and organ tissue is gradually lost with extreme caloric deprivation.

■ **Dehydration:** VLCDs, particularly if low in carbohydrate, can induce excessive diuresis, leading to decreased blood volume, which can lead to postural hypotension. Dehydration is potentially fatal.

■ **Ketosis:** VLCDs, particularly if low in carbohydrate, can cause ketosis. Ketosis is widely believed to cause euphoria and decreased appetite, although not all researchers agree. Ketosis can interfere with concentration and cause strong, unpleasant breath and body odor. In extreme cases may lower blood pH, which can be fatal. Ketosis is hazardous for pregnant women and insulin-dependent diabetics. Can be avoided if carbohydrate and calorie levels are high enough.

■ **Hypoglycemia:** VLCDs can result in excessively low levels of glucose in the blood, which may cause headaches, fatigue, inability to concentrate, sleepiness and cardiac arrhythmias.

■ **Hypokalemia:** VLCDs can result in excessively low levels of potassium in the blood, which may lead to cardiac arrhythmias.

■ **Hyperuricemia:** Excess uric acid levels have been caused by VLCDs. Gouty arthritis or uric acid kidney stones may be caused or exacerbated.

■ **Fibrosis of vital organs:** An abnormal increase in fibrous connective tissue in the organs may occur with repeated attempts at weight loss using starvation methods.

■ **Hair loss:** Hair loss is a well-documented side effect of VLCDs; usually temporary.

■ **Anemia:** VLCDs have been associated with anemia, characterized by fatigue, lassitude, weakness, pallor, reduced resistance to infection, lowered exercise tolerance and decreased attention span.

■ **Re-feeding edema:** With very low carbohydrate diets, large amounts of water may be retained when carbohydrates are consumed in a re-feeding process.

■ **Other documented side effects:** Included in other side effects are constipation or diarrhea, headaches, nausea, dry skin, gallstones, muscle cramps, bad breath, fatigue, cold intolerance, menstrual irregularities, and transient skin rash.

This statement was developed for the Michigan Health Council by a broad-based task force convened at the request of the Michigan Department of Public Health in response to "potentially-dangerous practices in the weight loss industry." It was written by Patricia K. Smith, MS nutrition candidate, Michigan State University, and Karen Petersmarck, MPH, RD, Project Director, Weight Loss Guidelines, Michigan Health Council. The recommendations are endorsed by 45 organizations and agencies. *Toward Safe Weight Loss: Recommendations for Adult Weight Loss Programs in Michigan.* Michigan Department of Public Health. *Obesity & Health Mar/Apr 1991;21-29.*

The biology of human starvation

Physical and personality changes in the Minnesota Experiment

Much critical information on the adverse effects of rapid weight loss can be found in Ancel Keys' classic 1950 book, *The Biology of Human Starvation.*

In this impressive two-volume 1,385-page work, Keys documents the physical and mental reactions of the 32 men who took part in the Minnesota Experiment in starvation of 1944-1945.

A well-educated and idealistic group, the volunteers were designated wartime conscientious objectors. All had at least one year of college; over half were college graduates.

Many had volunteered to serve overseas in relief operations. In participating in the starvation research, they hoped to make an important contribution to desperate people throughout the world. When the study began they expected to go overseas after the war to aid famine sufferers.

Unfortunately, their altruism disappeared during the starvation period and they became self-serving and wrapped up in their own concerns.

The study lasted one year: three months of an initial control period, six months of semi-starvation, and three months of re-feeding. Extensive testing was done at each stage and during the following year.

The semi-starvation diet, averaging 1,570 calories, was less than half the normal amount eaten during the control period. The volunteers were required to lose 19 to 28 percent of body weight, depending on body composition (an average of 24 percent). If weekly weight loss for an individual fell short of what was expected, bread and potatoes were decreased; if weight loss was too high, these foods were increased.

Physical activity was vigorous. Each week the men walked 22 miles, participated in 30 minutes of treadmill testing, and worked 15 hours in clerical or maintenance work. They also walked a distance to the dining hall, adding another two to three miles each day. This was continued throughout the study, however it is noted their work was done poorly during the final two months of semi-starvation.

As semi-starvation progressed, a great many physical and psychological changes were documented.

The following changes found in the Minnesota study may be similar to many which are experienced by persons engaged in other rapid weight loss efforts.

Physical changes

- Weight decreased an average of 24 percent, ranging from 18.8 to 29.3 percent (the men initially averaged 153 pounds, at 5-feet-10).
- Size decreased, especially in the diameter of upper thigh and upper arm where reduction was 25 percent; decrease in upper trunk breadth and depth, waist breadth and depth, pelvic depth, and neck breadth varied from about 9 to 15 percent.
- Heart volume decreased an average of about 20 percent; variability in heart volume was increased during starvation.
- Work output of heart per minute was reduced about 50 percent.
- Pulse rate slowed, from a mean of 56 initially to 37.8 beats per minute.
- Small decrease in body temperature.
- Veins were less prominent, and often collapsed when blood was drawn.
- Basal metabolism rate decreased by almost 40 percent by the end of 6 months of semi-starvation; metabolism was reduced per unit of tissue mass, as well as because of decreased size. This was calculated as equal to adaptive savings of 600 calories per day. (The researchers say some famine reports indicate women may have a greater decrease in metabolic rate than males, and also that women may have greater survival rates in times of starvation.)
- The men had an abnormal accumulation of fluid, which gave increased measurements for some in the ankle and wrist. (Edema is so closely related to semi-starvation that early terms linking the two were "hunger edema," "famine edema," and "war edema," writes Keys.)
- All the men felt cold and frequently complainted of cold hands and feet. Even in mid-July, they

wore jackets during the day and piled on blankets at night.

- The men felt weak and tired easily; voluntary movements became slower; their energy output decreased, even though regular physical activity was maintained including 20 miles of hiking per week.

- Their capacity to work decreased, especially that involving lifting, pushing and carrying loads. Also diminished was their ability to climb, walk long distances, and stand for long periods. Speed and accuracy were less impaired.

- Decrease in strength by about 30 percent in the forearm, legs and back.

- Decrease in endurance.

- Giddiness and momentary blackouts upon rising were common.

- Frequent reports of muscle cramp, soreness, and extremities that "went to sleep"; tendon reflexes were more sluggish.

- Frequency of urination.

- No increase in diarrhea, bloating, flatulence or colic such as has been observed in natural starvation areas.

- Sexual function and testes size was reduced. (It is noted that European famine reports frequently mention amenorrhea in women, impotence in men, delayed puberty in children, and decreased birth rate.)

- No impairment of visual ability was found, but there was an inability to focus, frequent eyeaches and spots before the eyes.

- Acuteness of hearing improved significantly, along with sensations of ringing in the head. Ordinary sounds were disturbing.

- Skin became pale, cold, dry, thin, scaly, rough, inelastic and marked with brownish pigmentation; skin ulcers and sores were common.

- Teeth and bones were apparently not demineralized as had been theorized; teeth were X-rayed at beginning and end, and decay was considered normal for a 6-month period. It is noted there is no evidence of teeth or bone deterioration from famine areas, and starving prisoners emerged from Japanese internment camps with teeth in remarkably good condition.

- Hair became thin, dry, and fell out.

- Senses of taste, smell and pressure seemed unaffected.

- The men appeared as if older, and behaved much older. They often said they felt old, but there were no indications of an accelerated aging process.

Personality changes

- Apathy, depression and tiredness increased.

- Irritability and moodiness increased.

- Self-discipline, mental alertness, comprehension and concentration decreased.

- Deterioration of spontaneous activity, including intellectual pursuits.

- Loss of ambition, a narrowing of interests.

- Feeling ineffective in daily living.

- The men felt distracted when they attempted to continue their cultural interests and studies. They were frustrated by the discrepancy between what they wanted to do and did do.

- They believed their judgment was impaired; however, tests showed this was unchanged, and they appeared to think clearly. (The researchers suggest this erroneous belief stemmed from feelings of apathy and narrowed interests).

- Decrease in sexual interest and loss of libido.

- Personal appearance and grooming deteriorated; the men often neglected to shave, brush their teeth, or comb their hair; they continued bathing, however, as one source of pleasure in feeling warm, and relieving aches, pain and fatigue.

- An average rise toward the neurotic end of profile.

- Six subjects reacted to semi-starvation stress with severe "character neurosis." Two cases bordering on psychosis included violence and hysteria.

- A rise in hysteria scores.

- Sensitivity to noise.

- Sometimes highly nervous, restless and anxious.
- The men carried out their chores and duties poorly.

Food preoccupation

- Increase in food interest; there was a preoccupation with food talk and food thoughts, though some subjects became annoyed by this in others.
- The men spent much time collecting recipes, studying cookbooks and menus, and fixing food saved from mealtime.
- An increased anticipation heightened their craving for food at meals.
- The men did much planning about how they would handle day's allottment of food.
- Food dislikes disappeared. Taste appeal of the monotonous meals increased as time went on.
- The men became possessive about their food.
- They demanded food and beverages be hot.
- They toyed with their food to make it seem like more and of greater variety. Often, toward the end, they would dawdle over a meal for two hours.
- For some there appeared a conflict in whether to stall out eating or ravenously gulp their food.
- The men became angry when they saw others wasting food.
- They ate their food to the last crumb and licked their plates.
- They did not dream of food, however, as some other reports have suggested.
- Extensive gum chewing; one man increased his gum chewing to 40 packs a day.
- Increased drinking of coffee and tea.
- The men increased their smoking, and some nonsmokers began smoking.
- Nail-biting, not seen in the initial control period, became common.
- The men became somewhat acquisitive in purchasing useless articles they could hardly afford and afterwards did not want; others became extremely anxious about saving money for "a rainy day."

Social activities

- Deterioration was seen in the group spirit. During initial 12-week control period a group feeling had developed which was lively, responsive, tolerant and happy, with outstanding qualities of humor and high spirits. This gradually disappeared, and the tone became sober, serious, and what humor remained tended to be sarcastic.
- The men became reluctant to make group decisions or to plan activities, even though earlier they had taken an active interest in making policies and rules.
- They were reluctant to participate in group activities, saying it was too much trouble to contend with other people; they spent more time alone, became self-centered and egocentric.
- Social interaction seemed stilted, and politeness artificial.
- Food was the central topic of conversation; the men of little but hunger, food, weight loss, and their "guinea pig" way of life.
- The men were aware of their hyper-irritability, but were not entirely able to control emotionally charged responses, outbursts of temper, periods of sulking, and violence. Some men became scapegoats and targets of aggression for rest.
- Occasionally, exhilaration and feelings of well-being were brought on by such things as a variation in daily routine, lasting from a few hours to several days, but these were inevitably followed by "low" periods.
- Educational programs, which the men had originally designed to prepare themselves for anticipated careers in foreign relief work, quietly collapsed.

Refeeding

For six weeks the men received varied calorie levels, from 1,877 to 4,158 calories, in four groups:

- The men's spirits continued low for six weeks, and many were more depressed and irritable than ever.
- There was a slump in morale, and the men lost all interest in their earlier humanitarian con-

cerns for the welfare of starving people.

- They became argumentative, and questioned the value of the experiment, as well as the competence of the researchers; they expressed feelings of being "let down." (This aggressiveness was seen by the researchers as evidence of increasing energy, and that the men were becoming less introverted and more interested in their environment.)

- Hunger pangs were reported as more intense than ever.

- During the first 12 weeks of rehabilitation, appetites were insatiable; all the men, including those on the highest calorie diets, wanted more food even when they were physically full.

- Many found it hard to stop eating, although "stuffed to bursting."

- The men were still concerned with food and their rations, above all else.

- They continued licking their plates, playing with food, and avoiding waste. Although this was a highly educated group, the men's table manners and eating habits had deteriorated, and during refeeding several deteriorated even more.

- The urgent desire for dietary freedom was so extreme that postponing it another week produced severe emotional crisis and nearly open rebellion. All were counting the hours until they would have more food, even those who been eating 4,014 calories a day for two weeks.

- During week 13, when restrictions were lifted, the men ate an average of 5,218 calories per day. Their time was largely devoted to eating and sleeping, and they ate nearly continuously, eating as many as three consecutive lunches.

- By week 15, there was more social behavior at meals.

- By week 15, the table manners of 19 of 26 men were normal or normal, but the other 7 still gobbled their food, had the desire to lick their plates and licked their knives when they could.

- Of 17 who left the laboratory, 15 reported they ate from 50 to 200 percent more than before the experiment and snacked often; one said he ate immense meals and then started snacking an hour after finishing a meal.

- By week 20, all said they felt nearly normal and were less preoccupied with food.

- By week 33, 10 of 14 who remained at the laboratory were eating normal amounts. The others ate more than before. One man, who ate 25 percent more and was gaining excess weight, tried to eat less but became so hungry he said he couldn't stand it and returned to excessive eating.

- Slowly humor, enthusiasm and sociability returned, and the men began looking forward to their plans for the future.

Physical effects in refeeding

- Physical discomforts continued, and the expected relief did not come quickly.

- The men gained fat tissue rapidly, and "soft roundness" became their dominant characteristic; in three months they had gained back an average of half their fat loss.

- Lean tissue recovered more slowly. Abdomin circumference reached 101 percent in three months for the highest calorie group, while arm, calf and thigh circumference recovered only 50 percent of initial size.

- The most rapid recovery was from dizziness, apathy and lethargy, with slower recovery from tiredness, weakness and loss of sex drive.

- Work capacity increased by week 13.

- The men had some problems with constipation, stomach pains, heartburn and gas, especially when they overate.

- Sleepiness and headaches increased for some.

- Thirst increased and edema continued to be a problem.

Source: Keys, Ancel, J Brozek, A Henschel, O Mickelsen, H Taylor. The Biology of Human Starvation. School of Public Health, 1950. University of Minnesota Press, Minneapolis, MN.

LONG-TERM BENEFITS AND ADVERSE EFFECTS OF WEIGHT LOSS: OBSERVATIONS FROM THE FRAMINGHAM HEART AND CARDIA STUDIES

Millicent Higgins, M.D., D.P.H., Ralph D'Agostino, William Kannel, Joan Pinsky, Janet Cobb, Diane Bild, and Phyliss Sholinsky

Identifying long-term benefits and adverse effects of weight loss is not an easy task, especially when they were not among the original goals of prospective studies of cardiovascular disease, such as Framingham and CARDIA. The emphasis in this conference is on voluntary weight loss and control whereas both voluntary and involuntary weight loss occur in free-living populations and contribute to the difficulty of separating causes from consequences and benefits from adverse effects.

Nevertheless, repeated measurements of weight, body mass index (BMI, k/m^2), and other measures of body size and fatness, together with measurements of mortality, morbidity, and risk factors, provide useful insights into the determinants and effects of changes in weight.

FRAMINGHAM HEART STUDY

Men and women ages 35 to 54 years at the fourth examination of the Framingham cohort were characterized with respect to BMI measured at 2-year intervals in exams 4 through 9, that is, over a period of 10 years. Individual slopes, based on regressions of BMI over this interval, were used to define three equal groups (tertiles) of individuals: those who lost weight, those whose weight remained relatively stable, and those who gained weight. Baseline characteristics of the three groups are shown in table 1. Men and women whose BMI's declined were older, heavier, and had higher systolic blood pressures and higher serum cholesterol levels at the beginning of the observation period (exam 4) than other men and women. Ten years later, they were lighter than the two other groups, and more of them were smokers. Their systolic blood pressures were higher at exam 9 than those of men and women whose BMI did not change but about the same as those persons who gained weight. Serum cholesterol levels were a little higher at exam 9 in women who lost weight, but they were lower in men who lost weight. When BMI and risk factor trends were compared over the 10-year intervals, those who lost weight had the smallest gains in systolic blood pressure and serum cholesterol and the lowest rates of stopping smoking.

Mortality rates from exam 9 to exam 18 (18 years of followup) were highest in those whose BMI declined during the preceding 10 years, beginning after about 1 year of followup in men, but not until after 6 years in younger women and 4 years in older women. In younger men, mortality rates were lowest for those whose BMI changed least whereas they were lowest in older men who gained weight. Death rates were about the same for the three

MILLICENT HIGGINS, M.D., D.P.H., ASSOCIATE DIRECTOR, EPIDEMIOLOGY AND BIOMETRY PROGRAM, NATIONAL HEART, LUNG, AND BLOOD INSTITUTE, BETHESDA, MARYLAND; NIH TECHNOLOGY ASSESSMENT CONFERENCE: METHODS FOR VOLUNTARY WEIGHT LOSS AND CONTROL, MARCH 30-APRIL 1, 1992

tertiles of BMI change in younger women during the first 6 years of followup, but they were lowest in those who gained weight after that. Among older women, mortality rates were similar in those who did not change and in those who increased in BMI.

Relative risks of dying from any cause are shown in table 2 for tertile 1 compared with tertile 2 and for tertile 3 compared with tertile 2. Deaths occurring in the first 4 years of followup were excluded in this analysis to reduce the influence of preexisting disease and to assess longer term effects of weight change. Weight loss was associated with increased mortality in men and women after adjusting for age and BMI at the beginning of the observation period.

CARDIA

CARDIA is the acronym for the study of Coronary Artery Risk Development in Young Adults. Black and white men and women were recruited at age 18 to 30 years and examined initially and again after 2 years and 5 years. Weights at the first two exams were used to define three groups: persons who lost 5 pounds or more, persons who gained 5 pounds or more, and persons whose weights were stable. Characteristics of these groups are shown in table 3.

The following statistically significant differences were found at baseline: women who subsequently lost weight were heavier, had lower levels of HDL cholesterol, and higher rates of cigarette smoking, initially. Women whose weight remained stable between exams 1 and 2 weighed least, were better educated, and less often on a diet, and a high percentage were white. Women who gained 5 pounds or more were also heavy at baseline, and a large percentage were black. Among men, weight loss was associated with being older and heavier and having higher levels of cholesterol and systolic and diastolic blood pressure but lower levels of HDL cholesterol at baseline. Levels of HDL cholesterol were highest and blood pressures lowest in men whose weight changed least.

To examine longer term associations between changes in weight and risk factors, those who lost weight were considered to have sustained weight loss if they did not regain 5 pounds or more by exam 3; those who gained between the first two exams were subdivided according to whether their subsequent weight gain was below (+) or above (++) the median for weight gain. No change in weight was defined as less than a 5-pound change in weight from exam 1 to exam 2 and weight gain of 5 pounds or less between exams 2 and 3. Changes in weight and risk factors over the 5-year interval between exams 1 and 3 are shown in figure 1. Mean changes in weight ranged from a loss of 15 pounds to a gain of 35 pounds in women and from a loss of 11 pounds to a gain of 30 pounds in men. Cholesterol and blood pressure changes were more beneficial in men and women whose weight decreased or remained the same than in those who gained weight. The pattern of HDL cholesterol changes was in the opposite direction but also consistent with improving or deteriorating cardiovascular risk as weight changes ranged from losses to substantial gains.

In summary, weight loss is associated with improvements in blood pressure and lipid risk factors in young and middle-aged men and women. However, cigarette smoking is associated with leanness and weight loss and may account, in part, for increased morbidity and mortality in those who lose weight.

Followup of middle-aged men and women in Framingham showed that weight loss and obesity were associated with increased mortality from all causes and cardiovascular causes.

Interpretation of the data requires consideration of age; sex; level of BMI; other risk factors, including smoking habits; and reasons for weight loss. Maintenance of stable weight and avoidance of obesity appear to be appropriate goals.

TABLE 1.--Means of Selected Measures by Tertile of Change in BMI From Exam 4 to 9 Among Framingham Women and Men Age 35 to 54 Years at Exam 4

	Women (N = 1,386) BMI change			Men (N = 1,114) BMI change		
	Loss	No change	Gain	Loss	No change	Gain
Age, exam 4	45.8	44.8	43.7	45.5	44.6	44.0
BMI, exam 4	25.8	24.0	24.8	27.0	26.1	25.7
BMI, exam 9	24.3	24.6	27.5	25.3	26.2	27.6
Men BMI, exams 4-9	25.1	24.2	26.0	26.2	26.2	26.7
SBP, exam 4	130.1	125.2	125.2	132.0	128.0	126.9
SBP, exam 9	135.3	132.6	136.7	135.7	135.0	136.5
SBP slope	0.5	0.8	1.2	0.3	0.6	1.0
% smokers, exam 4	46.0	42.4	45.5	64.5	52.2	66.6
% smokers, exam 9	44.6	37.0	38.5	54.9	44.9	42.6
Cholesterol, exam 4	240.9	229.1	222.5	237.6	234.5	231.0
Cholesterol, exam 9	248.1	247.2	245.4	228.5	234.8	234.4
Cholesterol slope	0.9	2.2	2.5	-0.8	0.3	0.7

NIH CONFERENCE 1992/HEALTHY WEIGHT JOURNAL(O&H)

TABLE 2.--Relative Risk of Total and Cardiovascular Mortality by Tertile of BMI Slope Ages 35 to 54, Exams 4 to 9, Followup Exams 11 to 19

Tertile of BMI slope	Men				Women			
	Age adjusted		Age, BMI adjusted		Age adjusted		Age, BMI adjusted	
Total mortality								
Loss	1.44	(1.14-1.81)	1.39	(1.11-1.76)	1.38	(1.06-1.81)	1.36	(1.03-1.79)
No change	1		1		1		1	
Gain	0.85	(.65-1.10)	0.85	(.66-1.11)	1.24	(.93-1.66)	1.23	(.92-1.79)
Cardiovascular mortality								
Loss	1.65	(1.16-2.33)	1.59	(1.11-2.26)	1.20	(.76-1.90)	1.11	(.69-1.76)
No change	1		1		1		1	
Gain	0.94	(.63-1.40)	0.95	(.64-1.42)	1.46	(.91-2.34)	1.37	(.85-2.21)

NIH CONFERENCE 1992/HEALTHY WEIGHT JOURNAL(O&H)

References

PART I
Chapter 1

1. CDC USHHS, Behavioral Risk Survey.
   Calorie Control Council, 1991 National Survey.
   Berg F; Who is dieting in the United States. HWJ/Obesity & Health May/Jun 1992:6:3:48-49.
2. Dieting and purging behavior in black and white high school students; JADA 1992;92:3:306-312.
   Adolescents dieting; JAMA 1991;266:2811-2812.
   Berg F; Harmful weight loss practices are widespread among adolescents. HWJ/Obesity & Health Jul/Aug 1992:6:4:69-72.
3. Berg F; Weight cycling: crash dieting drops metabolism for wrestlers; Wrestling with weight. HWJ/Obesity & Health Feb 1989;3:2:1-4.
   Steen S, and S McKinney. Nutrition assessment of college wrestlers, Phys. Sportsmed 1986;14:100-116.
   Tipton T, Physician and Sports-medicine. Jan 1987 15;1:160-70.
   Brandon J E, PhD, Differences in Self-reported eating and exercise behaviors and actual-ideal self-concept congruence between obese and nonobese individuals; Health Values May/Jun 1987;2:3:22-33.
   Int J Obesity 1985;9:4:257-266.
   Psychological Reports 1987;60:1151-1156.
4. Berg F; The weight loss industry. Regulation is needed. HWJ/Obesity & Health Jun 1990;4:6:41-46.
5. See 4.
6. Report of the Task Force on the treatment of obesity, 1991. Health and Welfare Canada.
7. Strategic Health Care Marketing.
   US Weight Loss & Diet Control Market.
   Berg F; Double-digit growth comes to abrupt halt. Recession hits weight loss industry. HWJ/Obesity & Health Jan/Feb 1992;6:1:8.
   U.S. Weight Loss/Diet Control Market, 1992, Marketdata Enterprises.
   Berg F; Meal replacement products show strongest growth in three market segments. HWJ/Obesity & Health Mar/Apr 1992;6:2:28-30.
8. Berg F; The weight loss industry; regulation is needed. HWJ/Obesity & Health Jun 1990;4:6:41-46.
   Berg F; The case against PPA; witnesses charge diet drug is hazardous. HWJ/Obesity & Health Jan/Feb 1991;5:1:9-12.
9. Petersmarck K, Smith P; Toward safe weight loss – recommendations for adult weight loss programs in Michigan, 1989. Michigan Health Council, Michigan Dept of Public Health.
   Berg F; Safety is the focus. Michigan sets guidelines for weight loss industry. HWJ/Obesity & Health Mar/Apr 1991;5:2:27-29.
10. Yang H, MD, PhD, Roth M, MD, Schoenfield L, MD and Marks J, MD; Risk factors for gallstone formation during rapid loss of weight. Digestive Diseases and Sciences 1992;37:6:912-18.
    Berg F; Nondiet movement gains strength. Thin mania strikes women, girls. Berg F; Thin mania turns up the pressure. Berg F; HWJ/Obesity & Health Sep/Oct 1992:6:5:82-90.
11. Keys, Ancel, J Brozek, A Henschel, O Mickelsen, H Taylor. Biology of human starvation. School Pub Hlth, 1950. U of Minn Press, Minneapolis, MN.
    J Amer Diet Assoc 1988;1:44-48.
    Berg F; Starvation stages in weight-loss patients similar to famine victims'.HWJ/Obesity & Health Apr 1989;3:4:27-30.
12. Petersmarck K, Smith P; See 9.
    Berg F; Exercising can be risky in certain conditions. HWJ/Obesity & Health Sep/Oct 1991;5:5:80.
13. Obesity Research 1993;1:1:51-56.
    Berg F; Linking gallstones with weight loss. HWJ/Obesity & Health May/Jun 1993;7:3:45.
14. Revised statement summary of 1992 NIH consensus conference on gallstones and laparoscopic cholecystectomy, Jan 6, 1993.
15. Wadden T, Blackburn G, Van Itallie T; Responsible and irresponsible use of VLCDs in the treatment of obesity. J Am Med Assoc Jan 5 1990;263:1:83-85.
    Berg F; VLCD specialists warn against hazards. HWJ/Obesity & Health Mar 1990:4:3:17.
16. Howard A, Howard Foundation Research, Cambridge, England, at the second European congress of obesity satellite conference on very low calorie diets in Cambridge in 1989. I J Obesity Nov 1989;13:2:1-9.
    Higher liquid protein death toll. JAMA 1978;240:140-141.
    The COMA REPORT Committee on Medical Aspects of food policy: the use of very low calorie diets in obesity. United Kingdom Dept of Health and Social Security Report 31, 1987, London: HMSO; as reported in I J Obesity 1989;13:2-6;190.
    JAMA 1990;263:1:83-84.
    Berg F; The COMA report – UK. The use of very low calorie diets in obesity. HWJ/Obesity & Health Mar 1990:4:3:22.
17. JAMA Jan 5 1990;263:1:83-85.
    Berg F; VLCD specialists warn against hazards. Berg F; 60 years of VLCD. Berg F; HWJ/Obesity & Health Mar 1990:4:3:17-23.
18. Berg F. Michigan sets guidelines for weight loss industry. HWJ/Obesity & Health Mar/Apr 1991;5:2:21-29.
19. Sjostrom L, Mortality of severely obese subjects. Am J Clin Nutr 1992;55:516S-23S.
20. Drenick E J, Fisler J S. Am J Surg 1988;155:720-6.
21. I J Obesity 1992;16:465-479.
    Berg F; SOS in Sweden. HWJ/Obesity & Health Nov/Dec 1992;6:6:103.
22. Welch T, Nidiffer M, Zager K, Lyerla R; Attributes and perceived body image of students seeking nutrition counseling at a university wellness program. J Am Diet Assoc 1992;92:609-611.
    Kano S, Making Peace with Food 1989. Harper Collins Pub., Scranton, PA.
    Wolf N, The Beauty Myth 1991. William Morrow, New York, NY.
    Clin Psych Rev 1991;11:729-780.
    Vitality. Nutrition Programs Unit, Health Services and Promotion, Health and Welfare Canada.
    Berg F; Nondiet movement gains strength. Berg F; Thin mania strikes women, girls. HWJObesity & Health Sep/Oct 1992;6:6:82-90.
23. Forse R A; Surgical management of obesity. Ernsberger P; Surgery risks outweigh its benefits. HWJObesity & Health Mar/Apr 1991;5:2:21-25.
    JAMA 1989;261:10:1491-1494.
    NIH Consensus Conference Mar 1991;32.
    Am J Clin Nutrition 1984;10:293-302.
    N E J Medicine 1984;310:352-356.
    Danish Medical Bulletin 1990;37:359-370.
    Neurology 1987;37:196-200.
    Surgery 1985;98:700-707.
    Mayo Clinic Proceedings 1986;61:287-291.
    Acta Medica Scandinavica Sup 1984;679:1-56.
24. Gallagher D, Heymsfield SB, Obesity is bad for the heart, but is weight loss always good? Obesity Research 1994;2:2:160-163.
25. Fisler JS. Cardiac effects in starvation

References for Obesity & Health are cited as HWJ/Obesity & Health (before title change to Healthy Weight Journal in May 1994).

and semistarvation diets. Am J Clin Nutr 1992;56:230S-234S.

26. Drenick EJ, Fisler JS. Sudden cardiac arrest in morbidly obese surgical patients unexplained after autopsy. Am J Surg 1988; 155:720-726.

SIDEBARS

S1. AP 1994;5:11.
   Berg F; Dexfenfluramine use risks brain damage. Healthy Weight Journal Jul/Aug 1994;8:4:66.

Chapter 2

1. I J Obesity Nov 1989;13:2:19.
   Berg F; VLCD specialists warn against hazards. HWJ/Obesity & Health Mar 1990;4:3:17-23.
2. See 1.
3. Petersmarck K, Smith P; Toward safe weight loss - recommendations for adult weight loss programs in Michigan, 1989. Michigan Health Council, Michigan Dept of Public Health.
   Berg F; Potential side effects of very low calorie diets. HWJ/Obesity & Health Mar 1990;4:3:21.
4. Berg F; Three companies charged with false, deceptive claims. HWJ/Obesity & Health Jan/Feb 1992;6:1:9,16.
   Berg F; FTC charges false claims. HWJ/Obesity & Health May/Jun 1993;7:3:47.
5. Keys, Ancel, et. al. The biology of human starvation. School of Public Health, 1950. University of Minnesota Press, Minneapolis, MN.
   Berg F; Starvation stages in weight loss patients similar to famine victims'. HWJ/Obesity & Health Apr 1989;3:4:27-30.
6. Shil, M, Olson J, Shike M, eds. Modern nutrition in health and diseases 1994:704. Lea & Febiger, Penn.
7. Berg F; Iron: a key to generating heat? HWJ/Obesity & Health Aug 1989;3:8:61.
8. Berg F; Thermogenesis and the thermal effect of food. Healthy Weight Journal Sep/Oct 1994;8:5:98-99.

SIDEBARS

S1. I J Obesity 1990 14:S2:147.
   Garrow J; VLCD destroys self initiative. HWJ/Obesity & Health Jul/Aug 1991;5:4:58.
S2. Bis Trib, Sept. 11, 1991.
   Berg F; 500 clients sue Nutr-System. HWJ/Obesity & Health Nov/Dec 1991;5:6:91.
S3. AP Feb 27, 1991.
   Berg F; Chinese puzzle. HWJ/Obesity & Health May/Jun 1991;5:3:48.

Chapter 3

1. JAMA 191;266:2811-2812.

Berg F; Harmful weight loss practices are widespread among adolescents. HWJ/Obesity & Health Jul/Aug 1992;6:4:69-72.
2. JADA 1992;92:3:306-312.
   Berg F; See 1
3. Kaplan Allan, and Paul Garfinkel. Medical issues and the Eating Disorders. 1993. Brunner/Mazel, New York.
4. Rosencrans K; Diet pills suspected in deaths. HWJ/Obesity & Health Jul/Aug 1994;8:4:68.
5. Wis Rapids Daily Trib Jan 27, 1994;5.
   Berg F; Ephedrine strikes again. Healthy Weight Journal 1995;9:1:5.
6. Berg F; Bee Pollen "cures" truckers of obesity, tumors, radiation. HWJ/Obesity & Health Mar/Apr 1991;5:2:30.
7. Rosencrans K; Diet pills suspected in deaths. Healthy Weight Journal July/Aug 1994;8:4:68.
8. Berg F; Feds act against mix of scams. Healthy Weight Journal Sep/Oct 1994;8:5:94.
9. Healthy People 2000, USDHHS, PHS, Sept. 1990;140.
10. Addictive Behaviors 2;1987.
    Int J Eat Disorders, May 1988;7:3:413-419.
    Berg F; 1990 health objectives on obesity. Berg F; Setting goals for the New Year and new decade. Berg F; Setting goals for 2000 A.D. HWJ/Obesity & Health Sep 1988:2:1:1-4.
11. See 10.
12. Williamson D, Anda R, Giovino G, Byers T, CDC, Madans J, Kleinman; Natl Ctr for Health Statistics; Weight gain caused by cessation of smoking. NEJM 1991;324:739-745.
    Berg F; Smokers who quit gain to average. HWJ/Obesity & Health Nov/Dec 1991;5:6:92.
13. Federal Register, Aug 8, 1991, 56:153:37792-37797.
    Berg F; FDA bans diet pill ingredients after nearly 20 years. HWJ/Obesity & Health Jan/Feb 1992;6:1:10-11.
14. Gastroenterology 1990;98:805-807.
    Berg F; Cal-Ban 3000 saga ends with raid on Florida offices. HWJ/Obesity & Health Nov/Dec 1990;4:11:95.

SIDEBARS

S1. Wis Rapids Daily Trib Jan 27, 1994;5.
   Berg F, Ephedrine strikes again. Healthy Weight Journal Jan/Feb 1995;9:1:5.
S2. J Consult Clin Psychol 1992;60:985-988. HWJ/Obesity & Health May/Jun 1993;7:3:47.

Chapter 4

1. JADA 1992;92:3:306-312.

Berg F; Harmful weight loss practices are widespread among adolescents. HWJ/Obesity & Health Jul/Aug 1992;6:4:69-72.
2. JAMA 191;266:2811-2812.
   Berg F; See 1.
3. Mehler, P and Weiner K; Frequently asked medical questions about eating disorder patients. Eating Disorders, 1994;2:1:22-30.
4. Kaplan A and Garfinkel P; Medical issues and the Eating Disorders. Brunner/Mazel, New York, 1993:101-122.
5. See 4.
6. See 1.
7. Mehler, P and Weiner K. See 3.
8. Baker D and A and Sansone R; Overview of eating disorders, 1994. NEDO.
9. See 4.
10. Berg F; Diet pill companies charged. Healthy Weight Journal Nov/Dec 1994;8:6:112.
11. Diabetes Care 1994;17:10:1186-1189.
    Berg F, Insulin withheld for weight loss. Healthy Weight Journal Jan/Feb 1995;9:1:5.
12. Kratina K. Exercise dependence. 1995.Eds: K King Helm, B Klawitte. Nutrition Therapy: Advanced counseling skills. In press.
13. Toward Safe Weight Loss - Recommendations for Adult Weight Loss Programs in Michigan. Center for Health Promotion, Michigan Department of Public Health.
    Berg F; Michigan sets guidelines for weight loss industry. HWJ/Obesity & Health Mar/Apr 1991;5:2:27-29.
    Berg F; Exercising can be risky in certain conditions. HWJ/OBesity & Health Sep/Oct 1991;5:5:80.

Chapter 5

1. Food and Nutrition Board, Institute of Medicine. Weighing the Options: Criteria for evaluating weight-management programs. 1995, National Academy Press, Washington, DC.
2. JAMA 1989;261:10:1491-1494. HWJ/Obesity & Health Mar/Apr 1991;5:2:23.
   I J Obesity 1993;17:453-457.
   Berg F; Surgery risks persist over time. HWJ/Obesity & Health 1993:7: 6:106.
3. Personal correspondence with F. Berg, Healthy Weight Journal.
4. Forse R A; Surgical management of obesity. HWJ/Obesity & Health Mar/Apr 1991:5:2:18-25.
   NIH Consensus Conference Mar 1991;32.
   Am J Clin Nutrition 1984;10:293-302.
   N E J Medicine 1984;310:352-356.
   Danish Medical Bulletin 1990;37:359-370.

Neurology 1987;37:196-200.
Surgery 1985;98:700-707.
Mayo Clinic Proceedings 1986;61:287-291.
Acta Medica Scandinavica Sup 1984;679:1-56.
JAMA 1989;261:10:1491-1494.

5. Surgery 1985;98:700-707, 1990;107:1:20-27.
Berg F; Surgical viewpoint. HWJ/Obesity & Health Mar/Apr 1991;5:2:18-25.

6. Draft panel statement, NIH, March 27, 1991.
Berg F; NIH endorses stomach surgery. HWJ/Obesity & Health May/Jun 1991;5:3:37.

7. Ernsberger P; Surgery risks outweigh its benefits. HWJ/Obesity & Health Mar/Apr 1991;:5:2:21-25.

8. I J Obesity 1994;18:2:14
Berg F; SOS studies continue in Sweden. Healthy Weight Journal 1994;8:6:106.

9. Food and Nutrition Board, Weighing the Options: Criteria for evaluating weight-management programs. 1995. National Academy Press, Washington DC.

10. Weight Loss Surgery Survivors SIG, PO Box 7441, Albuquerque, NM 87119-7441; 505-247-4359 KssNewMex@AOL.com.

11. Berg F; Surgical viewpoint. Forse R A; Surgical management of obesity. Ernsberger P; Surgery risks outweigh its benefits. HWJ/Obesity & Health Mar/Apr 1991;:5:2:21-25.Obesity & Health Mar/Apr 1991:18-25.

SIDEBARS
S1. FTC, Ofc Publi Affairs, Oct. 22, 1992.
Berg F, Liposuction ads. HWJ/Obesity & Health Mar/Apr 1992;6:2:23.

Chapter 6

1. Berning, J and Steen S; Sports Nutrition for the 90s. 1991:156-158. Aspen, Gaithersburg, MD.

2. Garner, D and Rosen L; Eating Disorders among Athletes. J Applied Sport Sci Research 1991;5:2:100-107.

3. AABA Newsletter Spring 1994:8
Berg F; Young girls victimized by 'skeleton' models. Healthy Weight Journal Jul/Aug 1994;8:4:64.
Berg F; The shrinking Olympic gymnast. Healthy Weight Journal Jul/Aug 1994;8:4:65.

4. Brownell, K, Steen S, Wilmore J; Weight regulation practices in athletes. Med Sci Sports and Exerc 1987;19:546-556.

5. Steen S, and S McKinney. Nutrition assessment of college wrestlers, Phys. Sportsmed 1986;14:100-116.
Berg F; Weight cycling: crash diet-

ing drops metabolism for wrestlers; Wrestling with weight. HWJ/Obesity & Health Feb 1989;3:2:1-4.

6. NYTimes June 18, 1991.

7. Wisconsin Interscholastic Athletic Association. Wisconsin wrestling minimum weight program. 1992. For more information contact: Don Herrmann, 41 Park Ridge Drive, PO Box 267, Stevens Point, WI 54481; 715-344-8580.

8. Tipton T, Physician and Sports-medicine. Jan 1987 15;1:160-70.

9. Berg F. High body fat brings early puberty. HWJ/Obesity & Health 1990;4:10:73-76.

Chapter 7

1. Berg F; Eating disorders - physical and mental effects. Healthy Weight Journal Mar/Apr 1995;9:2:27-30.

2. Brewerton, T; Sexual and physical assault are risk factors for bulimia nervosa. NEDO Newsletter 1994;17:4:1-5.

3. Fallon P, Katzman M, Wooley S, eds. Feminist Perspectives on Eating Disorders, 1994, Guilford Press, NY.

4. Baker D and A and Sansone R; Overview of eating disorders. 1994:1-10. NEDO, Ohio.

5. Reiff D, and Lampson Reiff K K; Eating Disorders, p31, 1992. Aspen, Gaithersburg, MD.

6. Sesan R.

7. Kaplan A and Garfinkel P; Medical issues and the Eating Disorders. 1993. Brunner/Mazel, New York.

8. See 5 and 7.

9. See 7.

10. Eating disorder profile: Nutrition Therapy in the Recovery Process. Golden Valley Health Center, Golden Valley, Minn.
HWJ/Obesity & Health Jul/Aug 1992;6:4:70-71.
See 5 and 2.

11. American Dietetic Association, Position of the Am. Dietetic Assoc: Nutrition intervention in the treatment of anorexia nervosa, bulimia nervosa, and binge eating. JADA, Aug 1994;94:8:902-907.

SIDEBARS
S1. Visser M, On having cake and Eating it. J of Gastronomy, Am Institute of Wine & Food 1993;7:1:13-14.
Healthy Weight Journal Mar/Apr 1995;9:1.

Chapter 8

1. Clin Psych Rev 1991;11:729-780.
Berg F; Nondiet movement gains strength. HWJ/Obesity & Health Sep/Oct 1992;6:5:85-90.

2. Keys, Ancel, J Brozek, A Henschel, O Mickelsen, H Taylor. The Biology of

Human Starvation. School of Public Health, 1950. University of Minnesota Press, Minneapolis, MN.

3. Turnbull, Colin. The mountain people. 1972, Simon and Schuster, NY.

4. Zuckerman et al.

5. Sagan, Carl and Ann Druyan, Shadows of Forgotten Ancestors. Ballantine Books, NY.

6. Wolf, Naomi, The Beauty Myth: How images of beauty are used against women. 1991, Morrow, New York.

7. Gabler, Neal, Entering the age of intolerance. LA Times 1/4/95.

Chapter 9

1. Timely statement. J Am Dietetic Assoc July 1989;7:975-976.
Berg F; Yo-yo dieting threatens heart; gain-lose-gain cycle may be as risky as staying obese. HWJ/Obesity & Health Nov/Dec 1991;5:6:93-94.
Berg F; Weight cycling: crash dieting droops metabolism for wrestlers; Wrestling with weight. HWJ/Obesity & Health Feb 1989;3:2:1-4.
Wadden T, Blackburn G, Van Itallie T; Responsible and irresponsible use of VLCDs in the treatment of obesity. J Am Med Assoc Jan 5 1990;263:1:83-85.
Petersmarck K, Smith P; Toward safe weight loss – recommended interim guidelines for adult weight loss programs in Michigan ,1989. Michigan Health Council, Michigan Dept of Public Health.
The COMA REPORT Committee on medical aspects of food policy: the use of very low calorie diets in obesity. United Kingdom Dept of Health and Social Security Report 31, 1987, London: HMSO; as reported in I J Obesity 1989;13:2:5-6, 13, 179, 190.
JAMA 1990;263:1:83-84.
Berg F; VLCD specialists warn against hazards. Berg F; 60 years of VLCD. HWJ/Obesity & Health Mar 1990;4:3:17-23.
Nelson Steen S, Oppliger R, Brownell R; Metabolic effects of repeated weight loss and regain in adolescent wrestlers. JAMA 1988;260:47-50.
Nelson Steen S, MS, RD and McKinney S, PhD, RD; Nutrition assessment of college wrestlers. Physician & Sportsmedicine 14:11:100-116.
Tipton C, PhD; Commentary: Physicians should advise wrestlers about weight loss. Physician and Sports Medicine; Jan 87:15:1:160-165, 166-70.

2. Brownell K and Rodin J; Medical, metabolic, and psychological effects of weight cycling. Arch Intern Med

1994;154;1325-1330.
3. See 2.
4. Lissner L, Odell P, D'Agostino D, Stokes J, Kreger B, Belanger A, Brownell K; Variability of body weight and health outcomes in the Framingham population. NEJM 1991;324:1839-44.
5. Nelson Steen S, Oppliger R, Brownell R; Metabolic effects of repeated weight loss and regain in adolescent wrestlers. JAMA 1988;260:47-50.
   Berg F; Weight cycling: crash dieting droops metabolism for wrestlers; Wrestling with weight. HWJ/Obesity & Health Feb 1989;3:2:1-4.
6. See 2.
7. Abstract, 34th Annual Conference on Cardiovascular Disease Epidemiology and Prevention, March 16-19, 1994; Healthy Weight Journal May/Jun 1994;52.
8. Abstract Am Soc Clin Nutr 1992; J Bone Mineral Res 1994;9:4:459-463; Healthy Weight Journal Sep/Oct 1994;8:5:86.
9. Foreyt J, et al; I J Eating Disorders, 1995, in press; Berg F; Weight fluctuation links to stress. Healthy Weight Journal Jan/Feb 1995;9:1:12.
10. Berdanier, Carolyn. Rat growth confounds weight cycling studies. HWJ/Obesity & Health Jul/Aug 1993;7:4:71.
11. Wing R; Weight cycling in humans: a review of the literature. Ann Behav Med 1992;14:2:113-119.
12. JAMA 1994;272;15:1196-1202
    Berg F; Weight loss campaign heats up. Healthy Weight Journal Jan/Feb 1995;9:1:11-12, 18-19.

SIDEBARS
S1. Am J Epidemiology 1989;129:2:312-318. Berf F, Weight cycling men. HWJ/Obesity & Health Sep 1990;4:9:65.
S2. Intl J Obesity 1990;14:4:303-310,373-383.
    Berg F, Weight cycling and WHR. HWJ/Obesity & Health Sep 1990;4:9:67.
S3. Obesity in Europe 88, 1989:55-59.
    Berg F, Weight cycling. HWJ/Obesity & Health Oct 1989;3:10:73.

Chapter 10

1. NIH Technology assessment conference: methods for voluntary weight loss and control, March 30-April 1, 1992.
2. See 1.
   Berg F; Methods for voluntary weight loss. HWJ/Obesity & Health May/Jun 1992;6:3:42.
3. Petersmarck, K. Does weight loss increase the risk of early mortality? If so, why? 1995. In press.

4. Cutter G R; Obesity and the implications of weight loss (Is there death after success?). Perspectives in Applied Nutr 1993;1(1):3-13.
5. Sours H E, Frattoli V P, Brand C D, Feldman R A, Forbes A L, Swanson R C, Paris A L; Sudden death associated with very low calorie weight reduction regimes. Am J Clin Nutr 1981;34:453-461.
6. Phinney S D; Weight cycling and cardiovascular risk in obese men and women (Letter). Am J Clin Nutr 1992;56:781-2.
7. Simopoulos A P; Omega-3 fatty acids in health and disease and in growth and development. Am J Clin Nutr 1991;54:438-463.
8. Berg F; Bone loss with weight loss. Healthy Weight Journal Sep/Oct 1994:8:5:85-86.
9. Bouchard C, Tremblay A, Despres J P, Nadeau A, Lupien P J, Theriault G, Dussault J, Moorjani S, Pinault S, Fournier G; The response to long-term overfeeding of identical twins. N E J M 1990;322(21):1477-82.
10. Van der Kooy K, Leenen R, Seidell J, Deurenberg P, Hautvast J G A J; Effect of a weight cycle on visceral fat accumulation. Am J Clin Nutr 1993;58:853-7.
11. Reed G, Hill J; Weight cycling: a review of the animal literature. Obesity Research 1993;1:392-402.

Chapter 11

1. Wolf N, The beauty myth: how images of beauty are used against women, 1991. Morrow, NY.
2. Kilbourne J; Still killing us softly: Advertising and the obsession with thinness. Fallon, P, Katzman M, Wooley S, edits; Feminist perspectives on eating disorders. 1994. Guilford Press, NY.
3. I J Eating Disorders 1992;11:1:85-89.
   Berg F; Thin mania turns up pressure. HWJ/Obesity & Health Sep/Oct 1992;6:5:83.
4. Eating Disorders 1993;1:1:52-61.
   Berg F; Television ads promote dieting. HWJ/Obesity & Health Nov/Dec 1993;7:6:106.
5. Newsweek Feb 1, 1993;64-65.
   Berg, F, Gaunt idols, HWJ/Obesity & Health Mar/Apr 1993;7:2:23.
6. Rothblum E. I'll die for the revoluton but don't ask me not to diet. 1994; 53-76. Fallon P, M Katzman, S Wooley, eds. Feminist perspectives on eating disorders. 1994. Guilford Press, NY.
7. Eating Disorders 1993:1:2:109-114.
   Berg, F; False media messages. HWJ/Obesity & Health Jan/Feb 1994;8:1:5.
8. JADA 1992;92:7:851-853.
   Berg, F; Kids fear being fat early. HWJ/Obesity & Health May/Jun

1993;7:3:46-47.
9. Food Nutr News 1993;65:1:4.
   Berg, F; Trouble ahead in disordered eating for kids. HWJ/Obesity & Health May/Jun 1993;7:3:47.
10. Reported from New Scientist by Am Anorexia/Bulimia Assoc Newsletter Spring 1994;8.
    Berg F; The shrinking Olympic gymnast. Healthy Weight Journal Jul/Aug 1994;8:4:65.
11. Tolman D, E Debold. Conflicts of body and image, 301-317. Fallon P, M Katzman, S Wooley, eds. Feminist perspectives on eating disorders. 1994. Guilford Press, NY.
12. Lyons P, D Burgard, Alternatives in obesity treatment. Fallon P, M Katzman, S Wooley, eds. Feminist perspectives on eating disorders. 1994;212-230. Guilford Press, NY.
13. Olson C, H Schumaker, B Yawn. Overweight women delay medical care. Arch Fam Med. 1994;3:888-892.
14. Sternhell C. We'll always be fat but fat can be fit. Ms, 1985.
15. Lyons P, and Burgard D; Great Shape: The First Fitness Guide for Large Women, 1988. Bull Publishing, PO Box 208, Palo Alto, CA 94302.
16. Clin Psych Rev 1991;11:729-780.
17. Berg F; Is prejudice real? HWJ/Obesity & Health Jan 1989;3:1:5-6.9.
18. Orbach S; Fat Is A Feminist Issue II.1982. Berkley Publishing, NY.

SIDEBARS
S1. Robinson B; Melpomene Report, Feb 1985:9-10. Melpomene Inst, Minneapolis, MN.
    Robinson B; Fashions in female figure. HWJ/Obesity & Health Aug 1990;4:8:61.
S2. McBride A, Overcoming Fear of Fat, p95, Harrington Park Press, 10 Alice Street, Binghamton, NY 13904.
S3. I J Eating Disorders 1992;11:1:85-89.
    Berg F, Thin mania turns up the pressure. HWJ/Obesity & Health Sep/Oct 1992;86:5:4.
S4. Dudley B R; Fat kills. Fat!So? (No.1). Fat!So?, Box 423464, San Francisco, CA 94142.

Chapter 12

1. Berg F; America gains weight. Healthy Weight Journal Nov/Dec 1994;8:6: 104-109.
2. I J Obesity 1989;13:2:1-200.
   Berg F; VLCD in brief. HWJ/Obesity & Health Feb 1990;4:2:12-13.
3. I J Obesity 1989;13:2:1-200.
   Berg F; VLCD in brief. HWJ/Obesity & Health Feb 1990;4:2:12-13.
4. A J Pub Health Jun 1988.
   Berg F; VLCD and obesity surgery after 5 years. HWJ/Obesity &

Health May 1989;3:5:33-38.

5. Wadden T A, Stunkard A, Liebschutz J; Three year follow-up of the treatment of obesity by very low calorie diet, behavior therapy, and their combination. J Consult Clin Psych 1988;56:6:925-928.

Berg F; Disappointing 3 year results follow combined VLCD treatment. HWJ/Obesity & Health May 1989;3:5:37.

6. Clin Psych Rev 1991;11:729-780.

Berg F; Nondiet movement gains strength. HWJ/Obesity & Health Sep/Oct 1992;6:5:85-90.

7. Berg F; Three companies charged with false, deceptive claims. HWJ/Obesity & Health Jan/Feb 1992;6:1:9,16.

Berg F; FTC charges false claims. HWJ/Obesity & Health May/Jun 1993;7:3:47.7.

Berg F; The weight loss industry. Regulation is needed. HWJ/Obesity & Health Jun 1990;4:6:41-46.

8. Federal Register, Aug 8, 1991, 56:37792-37797.

Berg F; Three companies charged with false, deceptive claims. HWJ/Obesity & Health Jan/Feb 1992;6:1:9-11.

SIDEBARS

S1. Hirsch J; Rockefeller Univesity, NY. American Journal of Clinical Nutrition 1994;60:613-616.

Hirsch J; Gropes in the dark. Healthy Weight Journal Jan/Feb 1995:9:1:16.

2. King A, A doctor's weight loss education. HWJ/Obesity & Health guest editorial Nov/Dec 1993:7:6:104.

3. Kumanyika S. Edpidemiologic Reviews 1987;9:46.

Kumanyika S. Obesity keeps scientists humble. HWJ/Obesity & Health May/Jun 1991:5:3:46.

PART II

Chapter 13

1. Eating and its disorders, Stunkard and Steller, 1984;1..

2. Andersen A. The last word. Eating Disorders 1994;2:1:81-82.

3. Bowers M. The Last Word. Eating Disorders 1994;2:4:375-377.

4. J Am Diet Assoc 1991 Suppl 91:9:A-152.

Berg F; Does dieting cause more harm than good? HWJ/Obesity & Health Nov/Dec 1991;5:6:94.

5. NAASO Sept 2-5, 1992 meeting.

Petersmarck K; Health risks of obesity and obesity treatment. HWJ/Obesity & Health Nov/Dec 1992;6:6:104-115.

6. NAASO. See 5.

7. Berg F; Nondiet movement gains strength. HWJ/Obesity & Health

Sep/Oct 1992;6:5:85-90.

Berg F, see 4.

Berg F; Who is dieting in the United States? HWJ/Obesity & Health May/Jun 1992;6:3:48-49.

Dieting and purging behavior in black and white high school students. JADA 1992;92:3:306-312.

JAMA 1991;266:2811-2812.

Berg F; Harmful weight loss practices are widespread among adolescents. HWJ/Obesity & Health Jul/Aug 1992;6:4:69-72.

8. Omichinski L; You count, calories don't. 1992. Hyperion Press, Hugs International, Box 102A, RR3, Portage la Prairie MB, Canada R1N 3A3. Winnipeg, MB, Canada.

Omichinski L; New frontiers in nondiet counseling. Healthy Weight Journal 1995;9:1:7-10.

Omichinski L; A paradigm shift from weight loss to healthy living. HWJ/Obesity & Health 1993;7:3:48-50.

9. Satter E; How to get your kids to eat - but not too much, and Child of mine. Bull Publishing, Palo Alto, CA. Satter Associates, 4226 Mandan Crescent, #50, Madison, WI 53711; 800-808-7976.

10. Hirschmann J, Munter C; When women stop hating their bodies. 1995, Overcoming overeating. 1988, Ballantine Books, New York.

11. Johnston G; New vision for exercise. HWJ/Obesity & Health Nov/Dec 1992;6:6:108.

12. Corporation professionnelle des dietetistes du Quebec, A/S Comite traitements de l'obesite, 1425, boul, Rene-Levesque Ouest, Bureau 703, Montreal, Quebec H3G 1T7 Canada.

13. See 12.

14. Berg F; Association for the health enrichment of large persons. HWJ/Obesity & Health Sep/Oct 1992; 6:5:90.

15. Promoting Health Weights: A discussion paper. October 1988. Health Services and Promotion Branch, National Health and Welfare, Ottawa, Ontario, Canada.

16. 1990 Health objectives for the nation. National health and nutrition examination survey II.

Chapter 14

1. Berg F; The weight loss industry: regulation is needed. HWJ/Obesity & Health Jun 1990; 4:6:41-46.

2. Petersmarck J, Smith P; Toward safe weight loss - recommendations for adult weight loss programs in Michigan, 1989. Michigan Health Council, Michigan Dept of Public Health.

3. Berg F; New York City takes a first step in industry regulation. HWJ/Obesity & Health May/Jun 1993;7:3:52-53, 59.

4. See 3.

5. See 3.

6. Berg F; New York State seeks new laws to regulate weight loss industry. HWJ/Obesity & Health Jul/Aug 1993;7:4:70.

7. New York State Assembly, Task Force on Food, Farm & Nutrition Policy, Albany, NY 12248 (518-455-5203; Fax: 518-455-5573).

Berg F. See 4.

8. Berg F; The consumer's right to know. HWJ/Obesity & Health Jul/Aug 1993;7:4:64

SIDEBARS

S1. Berg F; New York State seeks new laws to regulate weight loss industry. HWJ/Obesity & Health 1993; 7:4:70.

Chapter 15

1. Nichter M, Parker S, Nichter M; Body image and weight concerns among African American and white adolescent females: Differences which make a difference. Anthropology Dept., U of Arizona, Tucson.

Berg F; Beauty ideas are fluid. Healthy Weight Journal Mar/Apr 1995 ;9:2:26.

2. Am J Clin Nutr 1994:60:153-156.

Berg F; Is drug abuse the next miracle cure? Healthy Weight Journal Sep/Oct 1994:8:5:84.

3. Newsletter of the National Eating Disorders Organization (NEDO), April-May 1994:16: 7:3. NEDO, 445 E. Granville Rd., Worthington, OH 43085 (614-436-1112; fax 614-785-7471).

Levine M; 10 things men can do and be to help prevent eating disorders. Healthy Weight Journal Jan/Feb 1995 9:1:15.

SIDEBARS

S1. Nichter M, Park S , Nichter M; Body image and weight concerns among African American and white adolescent females: Differences which make a difference. Anthropology Dept., U of Arizona, Tucson.

Berg F; Beauty ideas are fluid. Healthy Weight Journal Mar/Apr 1995 ;9:2:26.

S2. Stimson K; NAAFA News, March 1992:6.

Stimson K; Boost self-esteem with fat affirmations. HWJ/Obesity & Health May/Jun 1993;7:3:56.

S3. News release, Healthy Weight Journal 1/15/95.

S4. Gresko R and Karlsen A. The Norwegian program for the primary, secondary and tertiary prevention of eating disorders. Eating Disorders 1994:2:1:57-63;

Berg F; Preventing eating disorders in Norway. Healthy Weight Journal Mar/Apr 1995;9:2:25.

Associations and resources

The following associations are involved with weight, eating behavior and body size. They have a variety of publications and materials available for health care providers, educators and consumers.

Eating disorders

American Anorexia/Bulimia Association
Regent Hospital
425 E 61st St, 6th Floor
New York, NY 10021
Tel 212-734-1114

American Psychiatric Association
1400 K St. NW
Washington, DC 20005
Tel 202-682-6138
Fax 202-789-2648

ANAD
National Association of Anorexia Nervosa & Associated Disorders
Box 7
Highland Park, IL 60035
Tel 708-831-3438

ANRED
Anorexia Nervosa & Related Eating Disorders
PO Box 5102
Eugene, OR 97405
Tel 503-344-1144

NEDO
Nationl Eating Disorders Organization
445 East Granville Road
Worthington, OH 43085
Tel 614-436-1112
Fax 614-785-7471

Eating

SSIB
Society for Study of Ingestive Behavior
Dept Psychiatry
Cornell University Medical Center
New York Hospital

21 Bloomingdale Road
White Plains, NY 10605
Tel 914-997-5974
Fax 914-997-5958

Size acceptance

AHELP
Association for the Health Enrichment of Large People
Joe McVoy
PO Drawer C
Radford, VA 24143
Tel 703-777-0800
Fax 703-777-6970

Ample Opportunity
Nancy Barron
PO Box 40621
Portland, OR 97240
Tel 503-245-1524

Council on Size & Weight Discrimination
Miriam Berg
PO Box 238
Columbia, MD 21044
Tel 914-679-9160
Fax 914-679-1209

DietBreakers
Mary Evans Young
Church Cott - Barford St.
Michael
Banbury, Oxon
England 0X15 OUA
Tel 0869-37070
Fax 0869-37177

Largely Positive
Carol Johnson
Box 17223
Glendale, WI 53217
Tel 414-964-2804
Fax 414-224-0243

NAAFA
National Association to Advance Fat Acceptance
Sally Smith, Director
PO Box 188620
Sacramento, CA 95818
Tel 916-558-6880
Fax 916-558-6881

Women at Large
Kathy Sandow
12 Chancery Lane
Hawthorndene, SA 5051
Australi

Obesity

Center for Child and Adolescent Obesity
Laurel Mellin, Director
Family & Community Med. & Ped.
Box 0900
University of California
SanFrancisco, CA 94143
Tel 415-476-1482

IASO
International Association for Study of Obesity
Stephan Rossner, Secretary
Karolinska Hospital
Box 605000
104 01 Stockholm
Sweden
Tel 46-8-729 20 00
Fax 46-8-33 0603

NAASO
North American Association for the Study of Obesity
David York, Secretary
Pennington Biomedical Research Center
6400 Perkins R
Baton Rouge, LA 70808
Tel 504-765-2548
Fax 504-765-2525

Index

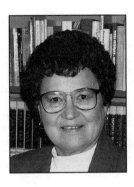

Frances M. Berg, M.S., is the founder, publisher and editor of *Healthy Weight Journal* (formerly Obesity & Health). A licensed nutritionist and family wellness specialist, she is the author of eight books. Berg's weekly health column, *Healthy Living,* has been published regularly in over 50 newspapers. She is Adjunct Professor at the University of North Dakota School of Medicine, Department of Community Medicine and Rural Health, Grand Forks. Her master's degree is in family social science and anthropology from the University of Minnesota.

Berg serves on the Boards of Directors of the American Diabetes Association, N.D. affiliate, and the West River Regional Medical Center. She is National Coordinator of the Task Force on Weight Loss Abuse, National Council Against Health Fraud, and a member of the North American Association for the Study of Obesity, the Society for the Study of Ingestive Behavior, and the Society for Nutrition Education.

"Timely, helpful, and thought-provoking. . ."
HEALTH RISKS OF WEIGHT LOSS

**SELECTED BY CHOICE, A.L.A., AS AN
"OUTSTANDING ACADEMIC BOOK OF THE YEAR"**

This first-rate report covers the scientific evidence on the health risks of weight loss interventions. It is about as far from the "hype and hope" that characterize weight loss advertisements as can be imagined.

The goal of the report, which is successfully achieved, is to educate both professionals and consumers about the complexities of losing weight, a serious matter with health ramifications that include problems ranging from gallstones to elevated cholesterol to death.

Above all, the report discusses the ethics of weight loss procedures in view of so much treatment failure and the harm that may follow from unskilled methods. The appendix includes, among other things, excerpts from the 1991 New York City investigation of the weight loss industry. References are complete and up-to-date.

Highly recommended to all general readers, all levels of undergraduate and graduate students, and the professional community.
— **CHOICE, AMERICAN LIBRARY ASSOCIATION**

This comprehensive report brings together for the first time information on the risks of dieting, weight loss surgery, diet pills, semi-starvation, rapid weight loss and the debate on whether to treat obesity at all.
— **BILL FABREY, AMPLE STUFF**

(Health Risks of Weight Loss) summarizes statistics suggesting few interventions currently used are successful, and none are risk-free. Potential side effects range from hair loss and anemia to increased risk of death . . . This book reviews the literature about the health risks of weight loss and concludes that the appropriate advice for many large persons may be to maintain a stable weight and avoid further weight gain.
— **JOURNAL OF THE AMERICAN DIETETIC ASSOCIATION**

Frances Berg, founder, publisher, and editor of Healthy Weight Journal, has compiled a comprehensive overview of provocative data that challenges the $30 billion per year weight loss industry right down to its foundation.

Scientific data from NIH conferences, the American Medical Association, epidemiologic studies, and Congressional hearings provide extensive evidence about the health risks of weight loss. These risks appear to be numerous, including life-threatening problems such as gallstones and cardiac disorders at one end of the continuum to dry skin and headaches at the other.

This book aims to help educators, health professionals, and laymen challenge widely accepted but potentially dangerous weight loss practices. The array of methods includes pills, surgery, exercise, starvation, purging, and a multitude of diets. Readers are encouraged to work toward the development of new intervention models based on more realistic attitudes, lifestyle changes, and scientifically sound practices.

Berg has compiled a valuable resource that acknowledges the complexity of the weight loss dilemma while calling for more humane and scientifically guided intervention. She has challenged current thinking and practice regarding weight loss while offering alternative directions for the future.

Highly recommended! If you are an obesity researcher, health care provider, educator or interested consumer, you will find this report timely, helpful and thought-provoking.

— **Journal of Nutrition Education**

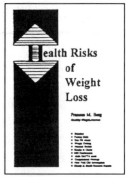

HEALTH RISKS OF WEIGHT
LOSS, THIRD EDITION
160 pages.

(Health Risks of Weight Loss) includes statistics which suggest a significant portion of the risks of obesity may well occur in its interventions, given the intense efforts made by obese individuals to lose weight. The book is intended to generate discussion that can lead to effective preventive action.

— DIABETES SPECTRUM

The report takes a strong stand in urging that obesity assume a high priority on this country's health agenda. The reality is that American medicine does not have an effective treatment for the myriad causes of obesity.

— ACADEMIC LIBRARY BOOK REVIEW

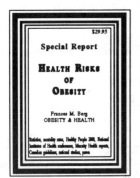

HEALTHY WEIGHT JOURNAL

keeps you current on the latest research

Worldwide, thousands of Healthy Weight Journal readers are learning
the latest and most accurate information on weight management,
diets, health, treatment and current issues.

"Your publication is the best – and I have subscribed to a lot."
- Jane Andrews, Registered Dietitian, Rochester, NY

*W*eight is a complex field, encompassing issues from anorexia to obesity.
You need to keep up on the latest research, but who has the time?

You do! Thanks to Healthy Weight Journal, the only publication to
compile and condense up-to-the minute facts and
figures on all aspects of weight.

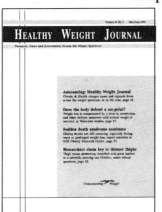

HEALTHY WEIGHT JOURNAL

is an easy-to-read update on weight issues from the fields of:

- Nutrition
- Medicine
- Public Health
- Exercise and Fitness
- Psychology
- Anthropology
- Family Sociology
- Child Development

HWJ cuts through false promises and quick-fix fads, gives you and your
clients a clear direction: good health at any size, not weight loss at any cost.
The answers you need are in each issue.

ORDER NOW to get the facts you need!

☑ **YES! I want to receive the top resources in the field
of healthy weight management. Please send me immediately the publications checked below:**

- ☐ **Health Risks of Weight Loss - $19.95 each**
- ☐ **Health Risks of Obesity - $29.95 each**
- ☐ **Healthy Weight Journal - $59.00/year (bimonthly)**

Quantity rates available on 5 or more copies

NAME --
(please print)

ADDRESS --

TELEPHONE --

POSTAGE: BOOKS: U.S.-$2.90 each;
foreign-$2.90 surface, $9.00 airmail.
SUBSCRIPTIONS: Canada, add $1.00 per
year; other foreign, $9.00.

Total Enclosed $_____

Method of payment *(US funds only):*
- ☐ Enclosed
- ☐ Bill me (Institutions only) PO#_____
- ☐ Charge card ☐ Visa ☐ MasterCard

_ _ _ _   _ _ _ _   _ _ _ _   _ _ _ _
Card number

Expiration date   Signature

CALL 701-567-2646 OR FAX TO 701-567-2602

OR MAIL TO: HEALTHY WEIGHT JOURNAL, 402 S. 14TH STREET, HETTINGER, ND 58639

**GUARANTEE: Your satisfaction
100% guaranteed or receive a
full refund, no questions asked.**